Alfred J.

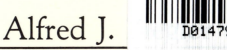

ARCHETYPAL MEDICINE

Translated from the German
by
Gary V. Hartman

with addenda translated by
Waltraud Bartscht and Carolyn Landry

Spring Publications, Inc.
Dallas, Texas

© 1983 by Spring Publications, Inc. All rights reserved
Reprinted 1985

Published by Spring Publications, Inc., P.O. Box 222069,
Dallas, Texas 75222
Printed in the United States of America by Edwards
Brothers, Inc.

International distributors:
Spring; Postfach; 8800 Thalwil; Switzerland
Japan Spring Sha, Inc.; 1–2–4, Nishisakaidani-Cho;
Ohharano, Nishikyo-Ku; Kyoto, 610–11, Japan
Element Books Ltd; Longmead Industrial Estate; Shaftesbury,
Dorset SP7 8PL; England

Library of Congress Cataloging in Publication Data

Ziegler, Alfred J.
　Archetypal medicine.

　Translation of: Morbismus.
　1. Medicine—Philosophy. 2. Diseases—Causes and
theories of causation. 3. Archetype (Psychology)
4. Medicine, Psychosomatic. I. Title [DNLM:
1. Psychosomatic medicine. WM 90 Z66m]
R723.Z5313 1983 　616'.001 　83-4757
ISBN 0-88214-322-0

Dedicated to our garden—where
the wind sings in the fir trees
and morning's dawning awakens
wonder. . .

ACKNOWLEDGMENTS

This book, except for the Addenda, is a complete translation by Gary V. Hartman of *Morbismus: von der Besten aller Gesundheiten*, published by Schweizer Spiegel Verlag, Raben Reihe, Rämistrasse 18, Zürich, 1979.

"Fever" was translated from the German by Waltraud Bartscht and appeared (in an earlier version) in *Dragonflies: Studies in Imaginal Psychology* 2/1 (1980): 36–46.

A former version of "Rheumatism: Of Joints and Stiffening" appeared as "Rheumatics and Stoics: An Approach to Illness through Archetypal Medicine," translated by Gary and Barbara Hartman in *Spring: An Annual of Archetypal Psychology and Jungian Thought* (1978): 19–28.

"On Pain and Punishment," translated by Gary V. Hartman, appeared first in *Spring: An Annual of Archetypal Psychology and Jungian Thought* (1982): 263–78.

"The Hydrolith: On Drinking and Dryness" was given first as a paper at the Eighth International Congress of the International Association for Analytical Psychology, San Francisco, September 1980. It was translated from the German by Carolyn Landry.

The three illustrations, printed on pages 8, 53, and 97, appeared in the Swiss edition of the book and are here reproduced with permission of the author and the publisher, Schweizer Spiegel Verlag.

CONTENTS

Translator's Note

There are always so many comments a translator could make about a translation that it is difficult to know where to begin. Often, though, the translator does best to keep silent and allow the completed work to speak for itself. This I will do with three exceptions: two having to do with the text itself and one a personal reflection.

Throughout the text, the term "empirical medicine" has been used to designate the traditional practice of medicine. The implication is of a perspective that follows a cause/effect thinking rather than the mercurial, "when/then" view of archetypal medicine.

Also, because language plays such a paramount role in archetypal medicine, I have, where necessary, sacrificed style in favor of a more literal translation. Some of the plays on words have perforce fallen through the linguistic cracks, while others have been added where contextually and etymologically possible and appropriate.

Finally, a personal note. This translation has taken two years to complete. To some extent this was avoidable, for which I apologize. A work of this significance and insight deserves to be available to as large a reading public as possible. To some extent, however, the length of time was dictated by the nature of the subject matter. Working through the material phrase by phrase, often word by word, I found myself dragged down, growing heavily inert, as if the concentrated focus on disease, death, and physical existence were exerting an enervating effect on me. At times I came to a complete stop and could not take up the manuscript again for months at a time. I came to realize that Alfred Ziegler has accomplished something relatively unusual: not only has he written *about* his subject, archetypal medicine, he has *practiced* it!

St. Louis
December 1982

Introduction

ARCHETYPAL medicine perceives medical reality according to a more or less definable theory, according to a particular attitude. Archetypal medicine's attitude or perspective, though, is no different from the attitude or perspective of the scientific/empirical healing arts insofar as each sees according to its own particular optic and can only be held responsible within the limitations of that optic. In many respects, therefore, archetypal medicine complements its scientific counterpart, completing to some extent, excluding to some extent.

Archetypal medicine does not depend as much on objectivity as upon subjectivity where the accent, in varying degrees, is clearly upon individual experience and its priority. It does not concern itself principally with the observation of symptoms but moves toward phenomenological amplification, toward the symbolic essence of what is observed. In the process, archetypal medicine turns up images which carry the symbolic essence and are accompanied by a perceptible physical resonance.

Far more than empirical medicine, archetypal medicine attends to the so-called "blood relationship," nourishing a certain intimacy and closeness. It is not so distant. As a result, medical reality does not as rapidly become a Cartesian *res extensa*, something strictly 'outer,' and the patient does not primarily become a kind of guinea pig. What informs archetypal medicine is not principally an admixture of sense perceptions with set categories to form constructs of pathology, technical functions, and abstract systems. Consequently, archetypal medicine must relinquish any claim to 'proof' for its concepts, since support for its theories does not stem principally from external evidence due to observation and mathematical/statistical acrobatics. It has recourse instead to 'inner' evidence, to understandings and certainties, enforcing them not with proofs but with examples which, compared to the tedium of statistical reasoning, seem more like play or a game. It occasionally cultivates the use of analogies, of the relationship among archetypal images, a pursuit reminiscent of magic.

The typological prerequisite for archetypal medicine does not lie as much in the capacity for registering sense perceptions—in extroverted sensation, in other words—as in the activity of subjectivity, of introverted intuition and an understanding of symbols. It requires a *cogitatio aurea*, a "golden" understanding, because "Habentibus symbolum transitus facilis est," "those with symbolic understanding have easy passage," according to an alchemical text. The maxim applies to medicine as well. Archetypal or symbolic understanding is also not an affair of the extroverted thinking function of intellectual manipulation but an *affaire de coeur*, of private feelings of universality which bring a particular harmony to all knowing.

The prerequisite for archetypal medicine is the very thing which causes modern behaviorism such insurmountable discomfiture: concepts resting on nothing more solid than thin air. These are concepts which have the effect of mere opinion, seemingly speculative, farfetched, or situational. They are only as valid as the number of those who profess to believe them. Archetypal medicine does not convince by experiments in a sandbox or, for that matter, in a Skinner box but by the experience of archetypal-image relationships arising from a kind of analogous intuiting. In no wise do the concepts of archetypal medicine approach those of scientific empiricism in clarity and exactitude. Rather, the boundaries are indistinct to the extent that we might well ask whether joining this with that can even be legitimate. The greater the claim to clarity and exactitude, however, the sooner a certain skepticism, even incomprehension, sets in.

Seeing in terms of relationships requires 'blinking' to make sight hazy. In archetypal medicine, seeing is not observing but perceiving, a perception similar to the mysticism of the Middle Ages' *cogitatio vespertina* 'the vision of twilight,' for analogies are not identities, and similarities are not equivalents. The difference is qualitative, not only quantitative, and necessitates a different kind of human being or a different kind of human seeing for this perception.

*

Not only the consideration of symbolic experience and the kinship of analogies within archetypal medicine suggest the spirit of sorcery but also the fact that everything presents itself in oppositions, as parts of polarities. It is as if the macro-conceptual, as well as the micro-conceptual, always conforms with closed systems so that every element becomes relative, something proportional. Validity converts to invalidity and vice versa. Above and below reverse themselves readily; health and suffering manifest changeable symptoms; the actual and the potential cannot be clearly distinguished. Suddenly the essential becomes the existential and pain, pleasure. Everything that happens can almost be considered a "Gestaltung, Umgestaltung, des ewigen Sinnes, ewige Unterhaltung" ("Formation, transformation, of meaning eternal, eternal diversion"), to borrow a line from Goethe.

The attitude is not as widespread in empirical medicine where pain is pain, body, body, and psyche, psyche. One is more likely to encounter the determined resolve to bring about a particular state denoting 'health.' Empirical medicine characterizes the situation as "serious, but not hopeless" and never as "hopeless, but not serious." Destinies become nightmares. Empirical medicine cherishes the belief that it—like the early church—carries the responsibility for the salvation of the fallen, no matter what the cost. It exemplifies our Zeitgeist, a thinking in terms of an *open-ended system* in which everything is irreplaceable, unique, and irretrievable, where obligations are at stake and action requires the teeth-clenching seriousness of heavy labor. While in empirical healing, tempers and arguments wax heated over conditions preceding the outbreak of an illness, conditions introduced by the meaningfully causal "because," archetypal medicine does not see causes but only conditions within a more noncommittal "when/then" framework.

Inasmuch as its perspective rests upon images and essences as well as upon opposites, archetypal medicine stems directly from the psychology of C. G. Jung, although the individual elements of Jung's psychology are not as relevant as the overall spirit of his thinking. One can hardly overlook the fact that Jung himself was of a mercurial nature and that Analytical (or "Jungian") Psychology, as well as archetypal medicine, approaches the realm of 'sorcery.' In both fields, for instance, reality tends to the sublime, to the half-real. Too, it was Jung's intuiting which led him from sense perceptions to essences, a process in which archetypal mythologems absorb the concrete realities, moving them into a dimension lacking something of earthly substantiality. In Analytical Psychology, things only have value within or as part of closed systems, existing primarily within oppositional polarities. But there exists yet another similarity between Jung's psychology and archetypal medicine's perspective: due to the relational thinking of both fields, perceiving through interactions of mystical marriages and separation, an *imago Dei* emerges which could be labeled mercurial/mystical.

*

Archetypal medicine is a type of psychosomatic medicine which attempts to bring about change in disease syndromes through language and, thereby, through reason. Despite the fundamental principles just described, archetypal medicine does not stop at reality's being nothing other than the cold, cruel, importunate world, nor does it ignore its pain. Rather, archetypal medicine counters any and all overly materialistic evaluations of the 'real' with a basic mistrust, a kind of *thanatropic irony* by and through which "the soul fallen into body" (to use a gnostic image) again bestirs itself. The most suitable medium for the process is *non-duplicitous language* with its hybrid nature. On the one hand, language has roots in the unequivocalness and factuality of physical reality and, on the other, it possesses a sublime quality which we call intellect. It is, therefore, mediator and magic wand par excellence, has a catalytic effect on every kind of all-too-material suffering, and provides archetypal medicine with the chance to loosen the stubborn restrictions of Nature—as have philosophy and religion from time immemorial. It is as if Nature had created a tool in language for preventing her own aggregate condition from becoming too pronounced.

Because archetypal medicine depends so much on intuition, a function whose perceptions occur in leaps, it cannot be presented systematically. Inasmuch as its nature is nonlinear, does not follow a logical progression but is, rather, intuitive, archetypal medicine can only be conveyed as illuminated parts, *luminosi*, in the hope that the parts might come together as broadly as possible as a collection of quasi-axiomatic images, a *galerie des tableaux*.

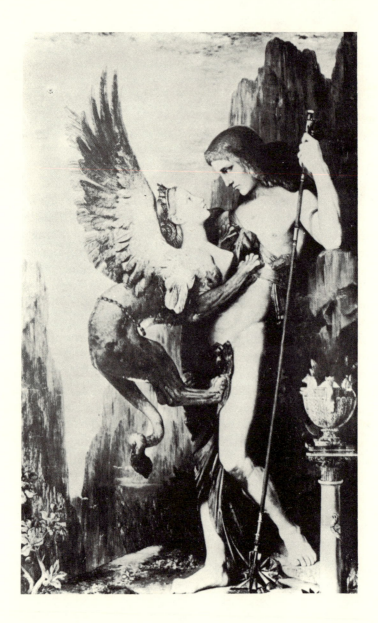

Oedipus and the Sphinx; Gustave Moreau. The destiny-laden
Greek was, himself, the chimera which laid in wait for him on
the road to Thebes to pose the question: "What is man?"

Theoria

MAN is a chimera, a monstrosity composed of an indeterminable number of contradictions. He is more of a monster than he is a rational being, a circumstance Nature has managed artfully to disguise to the extent that we feel more comfortable with him than we would with some bizarre creature from outer space. It is as if Oedipus himself were the very Sphinx he met on the way to Thebes who asked, "What is man?" It is as if the centaur whom the Greeks regarded as the ancestor of doctors already attested by means of his chimerical form to the truth that all essential knowledge about the nature of man has to be hybrid.

Or is it not true that in mankind love can be perverted to hate and the other way around, that efficiency carries slovenliness with it, or that behind all system and order the specter of disintegration shines through? Are we not confronted at every turn with the phenomena that paralyzing criticism glowers out of mother-love, that betrayal keeps the notion of fidelity alive and vice versa, that the fateful lot of the alcoholic stems from the insatiability of his sobriety, or that hypochondriacs expect the worst for themselves simply because they are so inconsiderate of their own needs?

Since psychology as a science, benumbed of spirit but rational in its approach, has grappled with existing conditions and phenomena, it has uncovered more and more such discrepancies. It seems, though, that psychology, upon discovering polarities—that extroversion and introversion intermingle in any individual, that a sadist lurks in every masochist, and that digital thinking must always be on the lookout for lapses into analogical superstition—rejoices unnecessarily. As enlightening as all knowledge of human opposites may be, our information to date is woefully meager. The entire wealth of human polarities seems only then to become visible when, in our brooding over the riddles of disease, we stumble upon the manifold human qualities which play such an important role in the genesis of malaise. Again and again a new polarity finds material reality, as when the conflict between submission and a stoic "No" comes to light in rheumatoid arthritis or when the discrepancy between a particularly dependent nature and a continually faltering intention to reject dependency manifests in multiple sclerosis.

Despite the fundamentally polar pattern, man's nature is not symmetrical; his characteristics are not arranged like the spokes on a wheel. Man is not a harmonic creation but has a definite profile and individual non-interchangeability. Poets have brought into being an immense abundance of these individual characteristics, while psychologists with their typologies cut very poor figures by comparison. There are the enlightened, the insidious, the fools; there are the upright who do right and shrink from no one, the direct, the roundabout, the crawlers, and many, many more. Yet, no matter what the contours, no matter what characterizes an individual as exemplary or revolting, we will discover that these characteristics are but the dominant, 'healthy' aspects within polarities, those traits which on a relatively consistent basis comprise the predominant personality and can more or less be relied upon. For the most part, the dominant traits assist us in making our way through life and in adapting to circumstances relative to our goals. These same traits are also the overvalued, glorified sides of our personalities within which the dark and unadmitted traits lie hidden, completing us as dichotomous chimeras. The dark traits would be the recessive, deceptive qualities of which we generally remain unaware and which alternatingly make their unexpected appearance. Because of their sheer unpredictability we find them irritable, especially when they get us into uncomfortable situations. Frequently, they are the very thing which calls into question the image we present for public consumption and which acts as the source of doubt of our own identity. The recessive traits are also the least adapted sides of our personalities, having finally a curious tendency to 'descend' into the body where they stubbornly clamor for our attention as disease syndromes. While the dominant, overvalued traits would lead us to view ourselves as the crown of creation, our recessive inferiorities provide us every reason to doubt such a conclusion.

*

Man draws his chimera-like nature from life itself, sharing this quality with everything that lives down to the most primitive organisms which trace their existence to the primeval ocean. Everywhere, not only among men, but among even the protozoa in the smallest puddle, life depends upon this chimerical nature, upon ubiquitously polar qualities. It devours in the abandon of an embrace; it is sensitive and immune to pain; it is heavy and light, bright and dim, pushes and is shoved, winds its way between health and suffering, swimmingly suspended with one part in the inorganic substance of its oceanic origins.

We could portray the beginning of life as a kind of primal, biological excrescence capable of separating itself from the surrounding, inorganic mother-liquor thanks only to the chimerical principle. It continued to grow, propagating itself in ever-new and unusual pairings. Had we come to earth from another planet and been unaccustomed to the multiform guises of Nature from earliest childhood, we would probably be caught up in wonderment at how much uniqueness was to be found in the realm we call our world. We would be even more surprised at the extent to which life seeks extraordinary balances, particularly at how this process preserves illness and death.

We would be wide of the mark to speak of protozoa as 'immortal' simply because they reproduce by division: they are as mortal as we are, swimming into toxic substances or blindly finding a gaping mouth and, hence, an end in some animal's digestive tract. Were this not the way of things, protozoan life would have increased wildly to the proportions of a nightmare. There is no immortality in Nature anymore than it belongs to the scheme of things for one-sided efficiency to be rewarded. Nature seems much more intent upon the creation of *bastards* in which the chimerical principle may best be preserved. In this way she fosters progeny from unrelated creatures in order best to fulfill her overall plan. Neither in the world of human beings nor that of animals does an accumulation of efficiency and health take first priority; rather the preservation of illness and death does. Darwin's visions regarding preservation of the species—and, hence, of life—are beginning to become a perspective of the past.

Seen from another perspective, that of death and the inorganic, life seems a kind of *emanation* from the mineral kingdom, a journey through unchartered swamps, or a balancing act. It is no mistake of Nature, but Nature's *plan*, that we fall, disintegrate, or dissolve—not only a foundering on the reefs of outer circumstances but also a well-programmed assortment of illnesses and deaths. The selection of diseases and deaths belongs to the chimera-like quality of human existence, while health as such is only a secondary concern.

*

We can regard illness as the transformation of recessive traits and tendencies into physical suffering. While they are inconsistent, capricious, and usually maladapted, these traits have the curious tendency to somatize and to appear as identifiable diseases, as *morbus*. What once we considered only 'behavior' or our 'condition' suddenly or gradually takes on physical dimensions and moves, in a manner of speaking, into another aggregate condition, metamorphosing us into 'cases,' bringing about our 'fall' from the realm of psychology into the realm of medicine. When teenagers, despite their upward and outward striving tendencies and the need to stand up to life and its demands, suffer from degeneration of the spinal column, do we not witness how humility and submission on a physical plane counteract the uncritical impudence of youth? Do we not see how the drive to inconsiderate domination of others is countered by a tendency to discretion when asthmatics are confronted with the new reality of having orders and insults catch in their bronchi?

The metamorphosis which results in physical disease is no autonomous act on the part of our deficiencies: illness is no isolated occurrence. Rather, it is brought about by a particular emphasis upon health, an emphasis which serves self-seductively in its compulsive and limiting nature. Somatization is inconceivable unless it is preceded by a 'going astray' of our particular talents. Nature seems to tolerate only a limited measure of one-sidedness—when the limits are exceeded or if too much energy is devoted to one-sidedness, Nature counterbalances the tendency through our bodies as if seeking a more effective or impressive means of demanding recognition for her chimerical plans. *The insensitivity of our healths determines our illnesses.* Our lack of concern and attention can only go so far before meeting set limits, limits which are difficult to determine but where one-sided superiority meets its opposite in physical form, where visible changes occur in the vertebrae and asthmatic constriction of the bronchi sets in. The metamorphosis or somatization itself cannot be predicted, although we may sense an impending occurrence of some sort, something 'in the wind.' Patients themselves are frequently unprepared, usually surprised by what happens to them. Questioning or introspection yields nothing concrete, while others can at least point to a hint, a suspicion of something which has found expression in reminders, well-intentioned advice, or frustration. Usually those who know the patient are just as surprised as he is by the illness, only wondering after the fact that something so obvious was not noticed earlier. Psychosomatic understanding is oftentimes from hindsight.

When Nature's plans, obscure as they are wise, achieve reality in an individual, the patient becomes akin to a baroque, sur-realistic figure. Among other things, the stricken individual awakens an entire spectrum of alienating feelings in others, for human nature harbors illness like a sort of perversion. Something strange or foreign, something that does not 'belong,' nests within illness. If the first, spectacular attacks of asthma shock us, if on seeing a painful case of poison-ivy rash we fall prey to the itch of curiosity, then the sight of a compound frac-ture can fill us with dread, and a watery-eyed cold can stir our empathy. With even a little sensitivity, we cannot help feeling that something absurd is at work, a feeling that our forefathers must have had when they described illness as the work of elves or of elfish lights, of beings somehow not quite human.

*

'The Fall,' the metamorphosis into physical suffering, is preceded by certain premonitions: Nature does not deal as underhandedly with us as it may sometimes seem. Long before the situation becomes serious from a medical point of view, our hearts are tortured with a hate which has only our best interests prophylactically 'at heart.' Long before any morphological changes are noticed in the spinal column of the hunchback-to-be, he is plagued by feelings of guilt. Long before the first asthmatic episode, nihilistic anxiety obtains, while actual diar-rheic crises serve but as the culmination of psychic incontinence in the face of difficulties. In other words, infarcts occur without actual infarcts, hunchbacks are not necessarily misshapen, asthmatics do not have to manifest bronchial congestion, and diarrhea does not depend upon the presence of frequent and loose bowel movements.

Nature may even be said to nurse the rich variety of these premonitory adversities, lending them at the same time a special measure of reality. Put somewhat differently, pre-morbid pre-monitions intrude just enough to show us where we stand and to what extent we have exceeded the natural limits of health according to a *law of intensity*, to degrees of priority. The fact that the premonitions are always present, in one way or another, bears witness to Nature's intention of continual prevention. Pre-morbid premonitions support health, precede disease, and guide those of us who pay attention on the path of physical well-being.

As long as what we have called "premonitions" remain barely perceived in a pre-morbid state, they may enhance our abilities to an extent undreamed of. They serve as a kind of leaven, motivating or driving us to escape into the ostentation of health and concomitantly outstanding performances. In this manner the pre-morbid premonitions fatten us up, a process which, thanks to not inconsiderable possibilities of repression and suppression, allows us to develop an unusually exaggerated image of ourselves. Even though the process can easily lead us astray and, thereby, evoke illness, it also provides us with the understanding for the very reverse, namely, how genius thrives in the dung of pre-morbidity.

In the long run, however, health undermines itself for, as our daily experience teaches, human life meets increasingly with disease and ends finally in death. We would have to be terribly naïve to regard Nature exclusively as having our well-being in mind: she does not work toward maintaining an eternally youthful state of health but toward our ultimate demise. Human existence fits Nature's plan only as long as it is transitory, and pre-morbid premonitions are not intended solely for prevention or as the hothouse for genius but much more as a *memento mori*.

*

Illness is our only heritage, for it requires but a glance at human life to determine that life ends in death by way of illness. It is only the spirit of our prospective, optimistic century which has forced this banal fact into the background of our awareness. We prefer to regard malaise as the doings of external noxae and aging as a breakdown due to wear and tear. Human life, though, does not merely wear out or run down; our heritage is not insufficient, defective, or eugenically inadequate. Our heritage, rather, includes *pre-programmed suicide* which determines the course of our existence despite all well-being and an amazing ability to hold out against inorganic tendencies. Despite all of life's vitality, we cannot ignore at least a minimum amount of inevitable decomposition.

Nature would appear to guard and supervise her intentions both jealously and mercifully, seeing to it that they reach fulfillment. Contrary to Darwin's liberalized developmental philosophy with its notion of the survival of the fittest, Nature eradicates especially the "fittest," thus asserting her principle of balance. Nature over-insures death. Should man succeed in avoiding the first trap she has laid, another just as certainly awaits him. Usually he carries numerous deaths around with him that stand in line for the opportunity to put an end to his existence. Life is not only "pathotropic" but also "thanatropic": its *telos* is not illness but death!

To this extent, man was conceived as a monstrosity from the very beginning; the monstrosity is not that he conceals deficiencies or shortcomings but is rather his chimerical nature. Man's heritage, his 'genes,' consist of 'dispositions,' of something, in other words, predisposed to dis-posal, to fall apart. Our inherited chimerical complements—dominant and recessive, superior and inferior—lend human existence its particular and unique characteristics. Despite all our fitness, our 'dispositions' subject us to the surrealistic transformations we call illness and, ultimately, to a unique and particular death.

We can grasp the original significance of the *Totentanz* images from the Middle Ages, images which generally portray those forms of human existence which Darwin would have considered "the fittest." We see not only voluptuous women with skeletal figures looking over their shoulders but also generals shaking hands with death one last time and burgomasters looking on as death lazily leafs through their papers. Human life, human existence, remains a dance of death, a *Totentanz*, because death is anchored in our genes.

Let there be no misunderstanding: the *Totentanz* in no wise epitomizes an exclusively wretched and painful condition. Death not only serves as malicious opponent or an insidious misfortune condemning the individual to a lifelong mésalliance, but also as "Goodman Death" he maintains long and intimate friendships. As we know from experience, there are those so enamored of death that they seldom emerge from their thanatropic infatuation. Their passionate liaison exemplifies what closer inspection reveals all around us—man possesses a primeval longing for inorganic existence and even a sense of regret that it ever occurred to Nature to bring forth something like life from the mineral realm in the first place.

Ancestors can pass on only a legacy of disease, their own dis-positions to disease, *not* specific illnesses. We do not inherit diseases as such but the predisposition to *be* diseased! Those syndromes which lend themselves most successfully to the efforts of psychosomatic treatment behave no differently than syndromes which do not. Those disorders allowing of the supposition that pathogenic factors are to be found among influences of early childhood (chronic arthritis, for example, or heart conditions) point equally as often to factors of inheritance, as do conditions on which psychosomatic medicine can shed no light at all. Twin studies, in particular, demonstrate these conclusions: they call into question all psycho-social attempts at prevention and deflate our cherished notions of attaining a disease-free utopia.

It has not been so long since man's relationship to death and the dead, including of course man's ancestors, was openly problematic. At the very least, there was cause for suspicion insofar as concern with death was not regarded as decidedly morbid or evil. Only with the advent of our positivistic and cosmetic century did we lose the habit of fearing the dead, having all we could do to deal with the future. Although feelings toward those who have gone before us are still problematic on deeper levels, we seldom deal with such things consciously. In highly industrialized nations, we seldom see the sick and crippled on the street, particularly when compared to the Middle Ages. Consequently, we are not confronted with the necessity for a 'more natural' relationship to suffering, mortality, death, and our own morbid natures. All of the cult practices which served to regulate and order relationships with the dead—and which prevented their intrusion into daily life with the resulting havoc—exist only as rudimentary remnants. Today, geneticists and eugenicists are the only ones dealing either ethically or medically with our unreasonably evil legacy. It is they who have undertaken to exorcise the dead, without being able to change in the slightest the basic nature of the disposition bequeathed to us.

Ethnologists suffer from much the same problem. Primal ancestors from which a totemistic society traces its lineage are characterized not only by unusual bravery, outstanding wisdom, and other positive qualities. Regarding the likeness of the revered ancestor as a totem figure or as a totem animal perched upon a post or pillar, the observer notices not only superhuman aspects but madness and disease as well. Everywhere the ethnologists uncover atavistic human monstrosities, genetic ancestral reversions, and disease. Here the goggle-eyes of Grave's disease, dental anomalies, dislocations, and compound fractures. There stunted growth or giantism, deformities, dermatoses, and symptoms which could easily be attributed to serious internal disorders. Hardly a single totemic figure exists which is incapable of evoking medical fantasies, a phenomenon which can scarcely be attributed to a lack of artistic talent. Artistic creations of primitive peoples seem rather to express a natural attitude of deep wisdom toward the morbid disposition of mankind, an attitude which finds expression in the masks employed by shamans for therapeutic purposes.

One might well imagine that a like sense of common ancestry underlies the formation of contemporary associations dedicated to this disease or that—the Lung Association, the Foundation for Multiple Sclerosis, or the Cancer Association. We can hardly overlook the importance of these groups but are forced to ask whether they really exist solely to promote the struggle against their respective disorders or whether they are not a manifestation of the totemic dynamic which binds all those together who suffer from the same disease?

*

While the dis-positions manifest themselves throughout an individual's life, they are less evident during childhood and youth, a time when heroic one-sidednesses, 'healths,' take form more rapidly than in later life. In the 'shadow' of these healths, however, stands the susceptibility to disease. Sören Kierkegaard, for example, was one of the first existentialists, that school of philosophy which placed especial emphasis upon *ex-istence*, from the Latin meaning 'to stand out.' One might well ask whether he would have been so effective as a philosopher had he not become hunchbacked as a concrete expression of doubt and humility?

That which becomes our strength in the course of normal development also provides the impetus toward sickness and death. In the process, the primal relationships of a child to his environment hardly deserve the privileged position generally accorded them by an age saturated with a product/causality mentality. It often seems as if there were relationships but no primal relationships. Dis-positions make use of an individual's environment throughout his entire lifetime—mother and father, siblings, house pets, and the chickens in the barnyard. Not only do parents and childhood environment have a formative effect on an individual, but they are also the first things that a child usurps!

Seeing the relative influence of childhood environment makes the wide variety of characteristics within the same family more understandable. Otherwise, the variability of personalities sharing similar origins bewilders and confuses: persons who are markedly different were spanked by the same father, intimidated by the same mother, consoled by the same dog, and awakened in the morning by the same pet rooster. Despite common environmental influences, each individual is molded by his respective disposition into unique, chimerical contours, finding his respective greatness and his respective recessiveness from which he sickens and dies. Kierkegaard's father probably misused his son's disposition to cultivate an existentialist philosophy: this same father carried a depressing sense of "silent despair" throughout his own life for once, while a shepherd, having mocked God for his low estate in life.

When our heroics, our special 'healths,' mislead themselves, our inferiorities and recessive qualities revert to bodily manifestations as *functiones minoris resistentiae*, functions with minimal resistance. Our shadows take on substance, ardently seeking out causes or things to cause their substantialization. The seeking appears to be so indiscriminate that it is satisfied with almost any 'thing,' perhaps one reason why disease was once regarded as a mania (for some 'thing'), a frantic searching causing one to waste away from his dis-easiness.

Suddenly aetiology changes from being a system of causality, a science which answers questions as to things and causes, to a system which describes the blind search for pathological noxae, therewith answering the question of the purposefulness, the *telos*, of disease in general. Both in the long and the short run, Nature needs disease to maintain her chimerical balance, grasping in her unpretentiousness whatever will serve her purpose: bacteria, viruses, fungi and protozoa, marriage partners, superiors or subordinates, automobile traffic, and the weather. Each of us has his own, unique murderer.

Imagine how different it would be to regard an individual suffering from allergic asthma as one experiencing the world as increasingly threatening, populated with growing numbers of spirits to the point that the most harmless objects turn into pathogenic parasites. It might be the dust on the table, an autumn mist, pollen, the smoke from the neighbor's chimney, an old acquaintance who is half-a-head taller, or even the sight of a vertical mountain face on a postcard. Man is extremely resourceful in his search for the necessary disease; the causes he simply conjures up out of thin air.

A long list of possible aetiological factors accompanies most disorders, awakening feelings of helplessness—as if one never properly understood the disorder without knowing the *real* causes. Both the feeling of helplessness and the assumptions as to 'reality' are justified. Yet, the lack of understanding lies not in ignorance of the causes but in the unnoticed arrogance of the notion of causality. To regard causality as the sole agent whereby definitive order can be achieved in the field of medicine seems to be both an inflated wish as well as a sign of the times.

From the perspective of archetypal medicine, *human environment is, from the very beginning, contaminated.* There exists nothing but pollutants since our dispositions are capable of converting anything into disease noxae. Our dispositions lend the "somatogenic" and "psychogenic" factors their effectiveness. Our environment is only as hygienic as the search for disease allows and, to put it bluntly, those who become concerned about air pollution are those who need it!

*

Contemporary notions of health and hygiene always tend to the classical, even classicistic: what the Greeks and Romans of antiquity depicted in their symmetrical, Apollonian sculptures differs little from our modern, conventional, amateur or professional concepts of health. It matters little whether the health be defined in positives or, as the World Health Organization does, in negatives—the WHO defining health as the absence of physical, mental, or social suffering. It is as if the goal of empirical medicine were the creation of Apollonian proportions and that the fate of the cultural historians during the last century still awaits medical science. As we know, the image of symmetry which scholars had created from antiquity underwent a transformation, thanks in no small measure to Nietzsche's *The Birth of Tragedy*. The beauty and harmony of Apollo discernible everywhere in Hellas (or so it was believed!) were joined by the disease of Dionysos, a god lacking symmetry in almost every respect. It seems that today we can hardly escape having to revise the classicism of medicine to bring it more in line with human reality.

Archetypal medicine's chimerical image of man is not classicistic! Rather, it becomes apparent that not only is there no such thing as a unified, indivisible 'health,' but also that at best there are a number of individual 'healths' which are identical with those dominants we spoke of earlier and which are particularly fitting in various respects. Accordingly, these 'healths' complement everything inferior or recessive and stand in a paradoxical attraction/repulsion relationship to all disease.

Just as there are but a limited number of diseases, so, too, should the 'healths' we are afflicted with be numbered—at least theoretically. The particular qualities of our 'healths' are actually only then apparent when we start from the diseases and extrapolate complementary qualities, qualities which otherwise remain for the most part indistinguishable in the shadows cast by consciousness's over-illumination. This is especially true for young people: since their concept of disease lacks concrete experience to lend it substance—is still nascent, so to speak—health correspondingly remains largely unconscious. Having been robbed or denied the experience of disease by our *Zeitgeist*, they know little about health and, by the same token, little specifically about themselves. Youth lives bewitched by the spell of its smooth, unsullied skin.

While Health moves and draws us upward—flies, after a manner of speaking—Disease moves heavily downward with its complaints, fatigue, paralysis, pain, and confinement (to bed, if nothing else!). In Disease we see helplessness and inactivity. In Disease we find the unhappy, the dependent, the handicapped. In Disease one writhes with pain or is immobilized by nausea. In our minds the entire process becomes idiotic as it becomes clinical, especially if we hear the Greek *kline* 'bed' in "clinic." Disease moves toward death as the condition becomes grave. We are mired down, pulled under, drowned. Progression is 'downhill,' down, into bed. One slip, one fall, and it may be some time before we get 'out' or 'over' it. At the same time, a sense of invulnerability accompanies disease: we are not confronted with any decisions, are not expected to come up with any solutions. We are exempted and suspended, the world has come to a halt, and we are, so to speak, dead, with the privilege of not being held responsible for anything.

Our inferiorities, our recessivenesses, acquire substance in our helpless, hopeless situations, calling us unequivocally to consciousness, a sort of re-minder that the uncertain balance of our health can take sudden turns. Our recessiveness regains significance during the heaviness of disease, scheming its own resurrection if it does not bring us once and for all into our graves. Those who have a curse catch in their throat due to a sudden asthma attack or those whose frigid desolation is warmed by a fever are given to understand in no uncertain terms that what hangs in the balance is not discretion or the warmth of human companionship respectively. Oftentimes, a skin rash is the sole means by which anger or love can find expression. Again and again, though, it seems to be the fool's gold of our superiorities, our dominants, which forces the transformation of complementary qualities into physical manifestations. Health always evokes disease whenever health becomes compulsive and is pursued ad absurdum.

To understand disease from this perspective, it is necessary to leave the firm ground of empirical medicine since, as experience has shown, categorizing pathologies according to disease entities does not allow for an appreciation of the mutual dynamic of health and disease. The diseases that we will be talking about are syndromes, *disease images*, not empirical constructs in which symptoms are more or less arbitrarily lumped together on the basis of statistical frequency and which, if possible, are linked to one particular causal agent. The disease images we will be dealing with are not intellectual formulations but rather graphic representations which appear in a most alienating, sensuous fashion.

Turning away from diseases as entities and toward diseases as images is almost an anachronism, a kind of medical regression to an epoch before rational, scientific research when diseases were spoken of in terms of images. It is as if archetypal medicine reverted to and sought connections in a time when one still spoke of colic, consumption, or of the "rose" as an erythema, to-day mentioned only as a symptom of dermatosis.

*

Diseases originate in abstraction. Nature cannot allow something so fundamental to the life process to depend upon the world of the concrete. Yet, diseases do not set in upon any *one* stage with a particular and familiar backdrop; rather they occur sometimes here, sometimes there, with little or no consideration for this or that environment.

If, indeed, allowing disease to happen belongs to Nature's intent or intentions, she finds the requisite 'causes' in the most disparate regions of the human world. Nature cannot afford the existence of 'healthy' living conditions: the Hottentot tribe in the rank, secretive, tropical rain forest lives no more dangerously than the population of an urban subdivision, and the taiga of the ice-ages concealed just as many (quantitatively if not qualitatively the same) dangers as does the contemporary world of industrial or corporate professions. Mankind's susceptibility to disease finds realization in the most widely varying circumstances and thanks to the widest variety of agents. In other words, military service provides as rich a palette of disease noxae as do marriages, families, job settings, clinics, hospitals, and—yes, last but not least—psychotherapeutic practices, for here, too, the sources and causes of disease are fervently sought after.

We see diseases arising more out of conditions which answer the question "how" than answer the question "what," more out of specifics and particulars. Diseases result less from particular behavior in association with particular objects as from the way and manner in which this behavior takes place, something essentially un-grasp-able. It is as if we had to relinquish all our concretism and had to forget the perceptions of our sense organs in order to arrive at that which contains the capacity of incorporation, an understanding or perspective on disease which platonically obviates an overemphasis on facts. We are dealing with an understanding which almost presupposes a reluctance to seek answers in the plethora of names, dates, and happenings pressing in upon us. Orientation can also be a form of blindness.

When, in other words, a stonemason suffers from eczema on his hands, it is not so much the contact with cement as an object or his particular activity as a mason which makes him ill. Rather, we would be justified in supposing the existence of an 'inflammatory' hyper-sensitivity to his trade made specific or qualified in a particular way by and through his eczema. Due to his sense of duty, the mason himself may hardly be conscious of his hyper-sensitivity. What is true for a stonemason is equally valid for a politician. The statesman who suffers a heart attack has not been endangered by politics and administration but by a hidden anxiety- and hate-filled despotism that, despite professions of a Christian sense of justice, somatizes and strangles his heart.

*

Disease demonstrates an insidious tendency to develop only to a particular degree of severity, as if the extent to which an afflicted individual's life will be threatened had been predetermined. The extent of somatization appears to be calculated, in other words, and the extent of the 'fall' into material manifestations of a particular form of behavior or state of mind apparently follows set laws of materialization. Chronic inflammation of the stomach, hyperacidic gastritis, cannot be expected to develop into a tumor as a matter of course, and simple headaches may remain simple headaches and need not change into migraines. Stiffness in a joint does not have to degenerate into rheumatoid arthritis, and a tendency to diarrhea by no means need mutate into an ulcerous intestinal infection. The opposite also holds true: just as a 'mild' condition does not necessarily degenerate into a severe one, neither does a severe condition 'improve' to become a milder one. Severe conditions are qualitatively different from mild ones and vice versa. In addition to uninterrupted transitions between degrees of severity, there are also graduated differences which Nature generally observes with exactitude. Organic medicine encounters here predictable phenomena similar to those found in Psychiatry. In Psychiatry, for instance, a neurosis does not presuppose an eventual psychosis, and even the so-called borderline cases remain borderline cases with considerable stubbornness, showing no inclination to assume the character either of a neurosis or to develop into an acute psychotic episode.

Conditions referred to as "mild" are much more *disturbances* rather than diseases per se and are termed "psychogenic" or "functional." They can seldom be reliably described or delineated, developing symptoms now here, now there. Along with constipation, for instance, one finds headaches or vague discomfort of the stomach or palpitations of the heart. Frequently, the complaints or symptoms disappear as suddenly as they appeared and are difficult to locate with any degree of exactitude. Sometimes they seem to be determined by environmental factors: symptoms occur regularly following this or that kind of experience or when preceded by a series of hardly registered wrongs. Correspondingly, their course is irregular, giving the impression of being arbitrary, even capricious. Complaints and symptoms lead us to false conclusions and to prescribing the most varied and wide-ranging of tests and examinations, occupying the attention of hospitals more completely, with their ephemeral qualities, than severe disorders. *Quoad vitam*, as far as life itself is concerned, these symptoms generally behave benignly, despite their capacity to terrorize like so many hobgoblins. Therapeutically, we often consider these patients candidates for psychotherapy, because the suffering appears to be 'nervous,' born out of and maintained by tormenting connections. For these conditions as for all forms of somatization, 'causes' or causal factors are usually but factors among other factors, tools in the hand of the disease instinct which utilizes whatever is most readily available to accomplish its ends.

In contrast to the 'mild' diseases, 'severe' diseases allow considerably more exact description. They do us the favor of behaving according to classic, textbook forms with corresponding progress and development. They appear 'statistically significant,' permitting a diagnosis under even cursory examination, and are the kinds of cases the medical novice believes he will be primarily concerned with. In reality, severe diseases—the cases a doctor can rely on and can count on as a part of his practice—form but a part of the whole area known as illness. The relationship between 'severe' diseases and the condition of the psyche plays such a minor role that seldom does the examining doctor even consider enquiring into the patient's job situation or investigating relationships within the patient's family. Severe diseases allow little room for caprice: generally they behave unimaginatively, sinisterly, autonomously, following some dark compulsion. Severe diseases are serious matters and need to be taken seriously, the extent of somatization reaching deep into the organism, right down to the bone, so to speak. It now becomes a matter of life and death, not simply a question of a greater or lesser amount of pain, nausea, diarrhea, and the like. Psychological therapy enters the picture only as a secondary

manifestation, illness, are in the final analysis necessary. Our daily afflictions are in no way solely an indictment of the *condition humaine* but an expression of satisfaction that our well-being and our human potential have boundaries at all. We are better grounded by the afflictions, protected and shielded, as if all our strivings assumed a touch of spontaneity. When we are short of breath due to obesity, we can take everything a little less seriously since we can, after a manner of speaking, hold fast to our own panting. Arthritic discomforts add a touch of pain to all our undertakings, legitimizing tendencies to indolence, while an acute or a chronic sinus condition enables us to hold the world at a distance with the excuse of "I have a cold."

As long as we know what to look for, we encounter examples of the law for the preservation of our 'undoing' and its corollary, the necessity of illness, on every corner of everyday life. When in the course of psychotherapeutic treatment the physical complaints or symptoms recede or disappear entirely, the circumstances and behavior which gave rise to the symptoms in the first place may well reappear as banal dysphorias. Where previously a persistent abdominal discomfort—with or without an accompanying bladder infection—complicated a housewife's daily routine considerably, now 'gripes' or complaints of a different sort confront her and make her life difficult. When, on the other hand, *psychic* difficulties take a welcome turn for the better, there is no guarantee that they will not, if they have not already, manifest as bodily complaints, 'fall into body'! When the suffering, the 'undoing,' expressed heretofore in stubborn and futile social protest suddenly improves, for instance, it would not be surprising to see it reappear as a painful abdominal rheumatism.

*

What holds true for the individual holds true as well for the collective. Nature has laid out a morbid world for us, intending our 'undoing' to be close to a probable mean and our state of health an approximate one. In other words Nature, even in regard to health and sickness, restricts herself to what can reasonably be expected of us.

The above perspective would probably find little favor in contemporary society. We might well be able to understand the necessity for a balance between births and deaths, lest we otherwise be confronted with the image of wildly metastasizing growth having eaten itself, literally, "out of house and home." We are far less able to recognize the homeostasis between health and disease. We might well acknowledge that a pond, undisturbed by human beings, comprises a closed, ecological system with a balance between what is healthy and what is ill, while we experience decided difficulty in regarding the world of human beings as the same sort of system conforming to the laws of illness and health. In this regard, we seem to be stuck in an ideology in which the spirit of positivistic scientism shines as brightly as it did during the previous century.

Nature strives toward zero population growth. Consequently, we ought not to consider genetic mutations in terms of those which are healthier as having the greater chance for survival and propagation. If Nature has produced something as specialized as cerebral tissue, she certainly has also had ample time to work out the considerably less complex process of the degeneration of the same tissue. Nature seems much more concerned that our susceptibility to disease and death keeps pace with all change and mutation, a consideration which seems highly plausible to us in terms of the animal and plant cycles of a forest clearing but rather odd and alienating when superimposed upon our own human landscape. To let go of our utopian notions and to turn to the realization that there ought not be such a thing as 'health' because there *cannot* be such a thing is at first glance disillusioning. We are hardly able to register the rightness and consolation, the somehow freeing quality of such a somber thought. Only, perhaps, in retrospect may it dawn on us to what extent our thinking is determined by the classicistic idea of

health, which only seems so clear and bright because its
motivating reasoning is so morbid.

Our health policies are at the same time just as exalted,
heroically as well as idiotically, if one perceives a thinking
behind them so emaciated as to be but a shadow of its former
self. The populace of Western nations represents a society that
in every respect has been corrected and polished to the point of
resembling a huge collection of restored, antique figures. Only
when one takes note of the number of people in a group who
have been surgically or chemically treated or in some way saved
from returning to the dust from which they came does one
become aware of the modern and yet never-changing ecological
intent of Nature.

*

Diseases socialize. It is difficult to tell to what extent all illness
makes possible the relatively peaceful coexistence within our
society. It would be decidedly one-sided were we to consider
only the difficulties and problems that confront us in diseases
and not consider the contributions.

We can hardly comprehend man's social qualities without
considering that man participates in society as a kind of chimerical nuisance: he shoves and is shoved, eats and is eaten. Society
is, for the most part, a viscous medium, and man's movement
within this medium requires considerable skill and energy. Activity in the human ecosystem shapes and molds our abilities
and talents, at the same time actualizing our morbid susceptibility, just as we humans for our part mortify and challenge our
environment. After a manner of speaking, society is a relatively
closed system in which we all have to find our places and in
which, not least of all, varying degrees of somatization play a
considerable stabilizing role.

In our human world, however, human beings are themselves
by no means the sole factor involved. Our world consists not
only of the species homo sapiens, no matter how ubiquitous it

might be. Within the medium wherein man moves—society in other words—man himself is but one quality among many, one part of a highly complex ambience consisting of much stone and concrete, artificial trappings, and bits of heaven, flora, and fauna. From at least the medical point of view, our fellow man has the same and equal importance as, for instance, one's house, the view of the mountains on the horizon, or the potted plant in the living room. Consequently, our sensitivities and apathies derive equally from and are directed equally at our pet cat or springtime with its pollen-laden breezes as at our fellows.

In particular as well as in general, morbidity or susceptibility to disease possesses a potential which should not be underestimated for maintaining social harmony, assisting in guaranteeing a highly hybrid sociability. Who knows how many marriages owe their existence to the migraine attacks with which a wife and mother grounds a crusty sadism and thereby saves the family as a whole? How many investigations have explored the extent to which an employer's feelings of hate and anger toward employees and customers find expression in the employer's heart condition rather than in poisoning relationships with other human beings? Who takes into consideration that the anxiety accompanying enterprising ambition often retreats into a susceptibility to attacks of diarrhea? Finally, how often have we recognized the importance of high blood pressure as a factor in stabilizing society, even preserving civilization to the extent that destructive tensions find a receptacle in physical hypertension?

It is conceivable that a given civilization would have greater recourse to such potentials the more it relied on an idealistic notion of harmony as an integral part of social existence. We cannot discount the role our so-called criminality and asociality play in this regard, nor the utility of our susceptibility to disease in embalming to a certain extent asocial tendencies in pathologies of different sorts. How many of us are aware of the positive implications for society of a disorder like arteriosclerosis to which the largest number of 'civilized' deaths are ascribed? How many 'attacks' of a physical, pathological nature were originally intended for others?

Our hospitals, then, assume something of a different role than the one customarily assigned to them: collection points for larval criminality. It would be worthwhile to investigate in each hospital ward how many broken bones had prevented a 'breaking' of the law. Clinics and hospitals honor in a fitting manner a form of criminal prevention which is seldom perceived as such and, because of the great amount of sacrificed antipathy assembled, they are transformed continually into a kind of *Hôtel de Dieu*. Certainly no one would conclude from looking at them that hospitals also serve as a kind of penitentiary.

*

Indeed, it seems to be those very contributions—be they political, theological, philosophical, or scientific—rewarded or motivated in a certain sense by pre-morbidity or disease which are of epoch-making or genial character. They seem to develop an even greater vitality and longevity the more they are rooted in a natural morbidity, the more they are embedded in Nature's paradox of health and disease.

This is one way of understanding the 'immortality' of the philosopher, Immanuel Kant, who is still quoted whenever discussions turn to the relative place of reason. As a member of the petit bourgeois, he strove to maintain a particularly 'reasonable' lifestyle down to the last detail. He never left the region of the city where he was born, living rather in terms of a strictly ordered space/time structure reminiscent of a prison. In his reflections on reason, space and time become the primary ordering principles according to which our relatively chaotic sensory impressions are structured. Kant's Enlightenment mind seems to have compulsively exaggerated the place of rationality, an irrational lack of reason which should have somatized as senile dementia. Actually, in his old age, a highly unreasonable spectral quality forced its way into his 'reason.' Or was it the case that this absence of reason motivated his philosophy from the very beginning as a pre-morbid backdrop?

What applies to the philosopher applies also to the scientist. Robert Mayer, for example, a doctor and theoretician, suffered from a manic-depressive psychosis, albeit one which did not conform completely with textbook examples. His disorder belongs properly to neurology since it is accompanied by a disturbance of enzyme metabolism in the cells of the brain. In his *Considerations on the Mechanical Equivalence of Heat*, Mayer proposed the law of the conservation of energy, an area which seems to have exerted considerable fascination for him. Would it be out of place to envision his epoch-making discovery as the concomitant of his physical condition? Would not the particular brilliance of his theoretical discovery almost have to be compensated for by some corresponding suffering?

Even political ideas have their origin in our organic nature. Rheumatologists investigating the pain associated with abdominal rheumatism discovered isometric muscle blocks serving to hold in check the superstitious belief in the value of an overly easygoing lifestyle. One can hardly help but transpose this particular example to a more universal sphere. It seems as though isometrically clenched fists raised themselves against any all-too-isotonic, democratic process, as if the dictatorship of the proletariat with an ideology tending to obstinacy epitomized the political equivalent of isometric muscular functioning.

*

Our Weltanschauungen arise from our organs. The human spirit owes its existence to them, being capable of thinking solely in the language of the organs and in such categories as provided by the viscera, the muscles, and the skeleton.

The brain is no exception, acting as but one organ among many that serve the intellectual/spiritual function. It provides only its own portion. An inspiration, for instance, is registered more often than not in the lungs, not in the brain. Psychosomatic medicine maintains a special reserve in relation to brain disorders, almost as if the brain bordered on the taboo, the realm of the ego itself, which as an Archimedean point had to remain inviolate. It is as if something in us rebelled at any attempt to relativize the ego or to involve it in a wider context. It is as if our very existence would be threatened by the notion that our brain with which we so closely identify might be subject to the very same laws as the stomach, the circulatory system, the genitals, or the musculature of the back. And yet the brain, too, is shaped by Nature much as are the viscera. It remains enmeshed in its dependence upon natural functions and carries out its singular activity much as does the indefatigable and stubborn heart. No matter what philosophical, political, theological, or scientific theories find their origins in us, the brain seems to play no greater part in their creation than the other organs.

The extent to which our organs determine our Weltanschauungen finds testament in our language. Any dealing with language and its history, with etymology, seems to lead to endosomatic sensations, sensations which then remain as the substance for all later formulations. Where etymology fails to penetrate to those sensations, it leaves the impression that its task is but half completed. If the so-called Indo-Germanic language roots, for instance, did not coincide with a physical sensation like *angh*, which surfaces in *angh*ina pectoris or in the German *Drang*, of *Sturm und Drang*, they would seem suspended, ungrounded, and rootless.

Even in those areas which are the most intellectual or spiritual, we cannot manage without the material of organic sensations. Just as our vision of the world is unmistakably bound to optical experience, so does every stance we assume in matters of the intellect rest finally in our legs. Under-stand-ing seems to have no more to do with our brains than with our other extremities. What is under-*stood* is correspondingly also something that becomes a matter of course and can be set or placed: it assumes a life of its own like the etymologically related "stool." Even that which is 'statistically' significant is something which can stand on its own and which we understand as a quasi-autonomous entity. When Martin Heidegger perceives the empirical world as a "stand" or framework, he intends a construct comprised of statistically meaningful building blocks, a philosophical stance which owes its existence to the legs on which we as human beings stand.

Wherever, then, do we obtain the notion that we are Nature's antagonists? Do not all the products of our technology carry the stamp of our organic nature? Is not technology but an enhancement or enrichment of Nature? Somehow we prefer to imagine ourselves as having escaped Nature or, at the very least, as having been banished or exiled by her.

*

While archetypal medicine characterizes a doctor's activity as "therapy," in those branches of the healing professions based on natural science the primary activity is "treatment." Whereas therapy in its original meaning implied 'cult,' the activity surrounding a disease, treatment is much more a mani-pulation, a laying on of hands with an authoritative demeanor. Treatment connotes a vertical relationship between doctor and patient by which recovery can be achieved.

Treatment is the logical, inevitable consequence of a Weltanschauung in which black is black and white is white, in which, as a matter of course, health and disease are clearly separated. In extreme instances, the perspective of treatment presupposes an unquestioned ideology in which disease, like some kind of misshapen surrealism, is measured against a norm of almost classical symmetry. Treatment presupposes a moral thinking and sensing as regards health and disease and for which health and disease are as distinct as angels and devils in the Christian perspective. Treatment draws continuing sustenance from a collective indignation over the evil in the world that only complete eradication could ever satisfy.

One can be certain that treatment does not perceive bronchial asthma as the suffering resulting when a tendency to expiratory brutality becomes inhibited by the fear of annihilation and which correspondingly deserves multiform condemnation. From the perspective of treatment, asthma is rather a respiratory disturbance, either mild or having a spectacular course, damaging, and clearly negative.

Treatment consists of a variety of techniques intended to restore a *status quo ante*, to return the patient to being "as good as new." Treatment consists of *countermeasures*, both surgical and chemical—in the case of asthma, in other words, of anti-asthmatic measures. Antiallergenics are prescribed, antiphlogistics, antispasmodics, antibiotics or, even, antidepressives. The basic posture is "anti," opposed to everything evil, in keeping with the principle of *contraria contrariis*. Treatment is antagonistic, with a view to restoring what was lost. Treatment is prudish, its efforts primarily apotropaic spells, exorcisms, and often fanatic persecution of disease. In like manner, treatment involves a form of hygiene which distances the patient from all possible allergens: carpets are wiped with damp rags to liberate them from malignant house dust. The effect reminds one of a kind of barnyard magic carried out in earlier times in the form of water lustrations. In addition we employ magical chants, incantations reminiscent of a purging or a kind of absolution. There is recourse to suggestive challenges and sobering appeals to be of good cheer. The doctor offers himself as a pillar of strength to which the hapless and hopeless patient can cling for support.

If the above portrayal of treatment sounds somewhat ironic, it is not aimed at treatment per se but at the medical notions that underlie treatment, notions which go so far as to lay claim to exclusive effectiveness. The sarcasm is directed at the seriousness with which medicine regards itself as the sole ethical position. The desirability of treatment cannot be questioned as long as life and well-being are of importance. Cynicism sets in, however, when medicine makes itself absolute and, admittedly or not, undertakes an exorcizing treatment which in its sadistic seriousness rivals the witch-hunts of the Middle Ages. Cynicism begins at the point where health and life—under the rubric of *salus est vita* (health is life)—are declared sacrosanct too much as a matter of course. Experience shows us how Nature undermines, with increasingly drastic measures, the drive toward health and wholeness the more obsessional it becomes. Sarcasm must set in before medicine's notions of itself become counterproductive.

*

While treatment primarily acts, the therapy of organic disturbances and diseases in archetypal medicine is verbal and extremely impractical. What activity there is consists only of certain 'cult-like' gestures and mimic directives designed to complement the focus on the verbal.

Yet verbal therapy does not deal in jargon and incantations, nor does it parcel out advice. No particular claims to authority are made. Therapy remains a dialogue, striving continually toward the horizontal relationship between patient and therapist. In principle, therapy would correspondingly require a minimum of technical know-how and that much more empathy and an ever-watchful, scintillating creativity to thread a way through the vicissitudes of conflicts and paradoxes. Instead of enterprise and rationality, therapy allies itself more readily with mercurial spirit, which timelessly leads and misleads. Through dialectic, therapy strives to come to terms with the complementarity of all disparate tendencies.

Whereas treatment lives on the strict differentiation between black and white, health and disease, the therapeutic aspects of archetypal medicine lie in a mystical twilight in which oppositionalisms realize their related connections. It is a form of medicine in which positions constantly change, where now the sick becomes the well, now the well the sick. Sometimes it seems that the capacity for the well to become the sick were the sole healthy factor, that a patient's health were but a questionable form of morbidity.

Being relational or relative, therapy in archetypal medicine is freer of moral overtones than is treatment. Therapy is not as subject to the Damoclean search for past failures nor to the spirit of a worship of life and health. In therapy, disease is far less a work of the Devil waiting to be eradicated. Should he appear nevertheless, then he usually does so as "jene Kraft, die stets das Boese will, und stets das Gute schafft" ("that power that always intends evil and accomplishes good"). Even the horror accompanying him can often be perceived as a Luciferian twilight. Medical cynicism, which flourishes all the more the more widespread the obligations of the Hippocratic oath, appears as a mild irony. Thus the therapy of archetypal medicine which deals with human beings as chimerical objects is related to alchemy. Archetypal medicine, too, is an art of gold- and dung-making, where treasure is found in gutter sewage or gold transforms into ram's dung, depending on the relevancies set by Nature.

*

Primarily out of trust in the alliance with the 'Devil,' archetypal medicine's verbal therapy seeks to 'redeem' that which has metamorphosed into physical disease. We can envision the process as a 'resublimation' of something that has fallen victim to materialization. *Sublim* can be understood as 'floating,' a complementary condition to that which in Latin is designated *gravis* ('heavy,' 'severe') and, in English, "gravitation."

Precisely by means of its almost ironic, quasi-masochistic position toward disease, its tendency to a mystique of suffering, and its love relationship—bordering on the perverse—with illness, archetypal medicine attempts to draw spirit from matter. The process does not occur without a kind of *Todeshochzeit* (marriage with death). Suppose the asthmatic became aware that Nature intended to strangle him because of his leanings to expiratory grandeur. Then it might also occur to him that his inner suffocation could only be lifted out of the physical realm when suffocation in the form of self-limitation enters into a liaison with his tendencies to 'greatness.' He may realize that he has no choice but to 'marry' the monster, to enter upon a *Todeshochzeit*. The term is perhaps a bit grandiloquent but certainly applies. Furthermore, it evokes the general mythologem of something particularly desirable joining with something dreadful and, thereby, 'dying'—a monster containing something of hidden value. A *Todeshochzeit* is only superficially such since death plays but a very minor actual role and then only from a distance. Usually it is but the specter of the *Todeshochzeit* which arouses horror, disbelief, laughter, or indignation.

The unusual conjunction with 'death' results in a sense of expanding horizons—as if the sufferer experienced 'eternity.' It is as if the individual's life for the first time acquired unmistakable and incorruptible uniqueness, particular limitation and freedom simultaneously. It is as if this recognition conferred an unassailable security amid the hustle and bustle of human existence.

The moment of this 'mystical marriage' may also carry bliss or ecstasy with it. Just as eternity is not solely a realm we enter at the close of our lives, an empire in which the ravages of time no longer affect us, so is ecstasy not solely a condition which begins with eternity. Ecstasy may occur with every marriage. Certainly not the least of marriages would be the *Todeshochzeit*, as long as we do not understand ecstasy as a euphoric exuberance but rather as an inner sense of security and well-being. The terms we usually associate with religion reoccur in medicine in conjunction with the manner and form in which we experience health and disease.

What applies to eternity and eternal ecstasy applies to 'resurrection' as well. We need not understand resurrection exclusively as a posthumous ascent of an astral body. That is but the religious version of a completely realistic event, what medicine refers to as "reconvalescence." Whenever life continues following those experiences we have called *Todeshochzeit*, something akin to a resurrection has taken place. When an infarct patient's condition improves after he has been released from the sinister *machine infernale* of an intensive care unit, he shows all the signs of having experienced a *Todeshochzeit*. He may resolve no longer to invest so much 'heart' in things once felt to be important— until an unheeded hate literally attacks him. If he adopts the perhaps naïve-seeming attitude of not taking things so seriously anymore, he is headed for a *status quo ante*, albeit one in which a certain reserve has taken its place. Reconvalescence, in other words, is a reconstituting in which we take something previously regarded as unworthy or useless and join with it in a kind of sacramental marriage.

Reconvalescence, therefore, resembles those resurrection images of Christian origin in which the resurrected Christ is afflicted with all the signs of his recent agonizing ordeal. The risen Christ of Grunewald's "Isenheim Altarpiece" emanates not only a sense of the eternal as He hovers before the backdrop of the universe, not only a sense of ecstasy as illumination transforms the materiality of His body into something pneumatic. Rather, He carries also the marks of his wounds emitting a phosphorescent glow surpassing all profane, first aid/emergency surgery. Christ appears like the martyrs of Christianity in general. Charity and piety, belief in a hereafter and eternal peace, and a condemnation of all brutality force brutality to realize itself in martyrs physically. Correspondingly, saints are, as a rule, mutilated. Had they perceived their existence from a less idealistic, more morbid point of view, they would probably not as often have found such glorious and heroic ends.

*

It is as if human beings moved throughout their lives up and down on a vertical axis only finally to end and remain at the bottom. The conditions we term "reconvalescence," recovery, and remission belong to this image under the rubric of relapse. It is as if all of life's uncertainty were an expression of the same truth, namely, that life is a hovering over the abyss of death.

The course reconvalescence takes is not only noticeable within the framework of verbal therapy. Left to itself or under treatment, the basic condition generally improves, but slowly and then interrupted by relapses. The lucid intervals last longer, the relapses become less serious and lose the character of the aporetical, the hopeless, the total. Particularly then, however, when the old attitudes reassert themselves too rapidly and the prior, superficially healthy one-sidedness takes over as if nothing had happened, they readily undermine themselves all over again. Reconvalescence is a sort of reflective image for Nature's tendency to allow our chimerical existence to disintegrate cascade-like in a series of ever-descending steps. It is the reverse of the life pattern, according to which we recover after each more or less serious fall, only finally still to arrive at death. *We are all chronic patients* who from time to time get better.

This principle applies to most diseases. A case of flu may seem almost comical in young people, its insidious nature only then becoming apparent when an elderly individual is stricken. Although varicose veins may strike us as mere cosmetic annoyances, they may give rise to thrombosis or to an embolic syndrome leading later to death. Every sickbed takes on an agonal quality as if every patient were laid out on his death bed.

*

Archetypal medicine portrays bodily suffering in the form of materialization and resublimation due to overextended one-sidedness. In religious imagery, archetypal medicine finds a connection to an age-old tradition, although religious perspectives are maintained less by mystical equanimity and esoteric irony and more by moral sensibilities. What archetypal medicine regards as a homeostatic play of uncreated creation religion sees as a serious, even grim, struggle for power. Consequently, religion's terms are not quasi-physical but stem directly from moral philosophy: sin, chastisement, and atonement.

Religious moralizing is not a phenomenon we have outgrown nor does it apply only to the preserve of a few sects. A moralistic sense for one's own disease is present at least to some extent in even the most enlightened. Usually, disease is no longer perceived as a shadowy struggle with an offended god or an insulted demon. Rather, remorse or regret sets in when, after the fact, the correlation between a disease or chronic suffering and our lifestyle—something which might have been avoided— becomes apparent. Moral overtones resonate even today in all pathology: responsibility, guilt, punishment, and atonement. In earlier times, such a moralistic perspective of disease stood in relation to socializing norms and to an individual's connection to the divine. Human hubris, blasphemy against divine order, sacrilegious swearing, and malice toward all that a god had created drew down disease as punishment. The model is not only Christian but generally religious and ubiquitous, a primal image of how man perceives the coming and going of disease.

Not only is it the Christian devil who limps about like an orthopedic patient, who was thrown from heaven to earth because of his opposition to God's plan for salvation: in like manner was the Greeks' Hephaistos cast down from Mount Olympus. Prometheus, who stole fire from Olympus for mankind because he could not bear their misery, was chained by Zeus to a rock in the Caucasus where an eagle ate out his liver by day only for it to grow back by night. His wantonness was followed by the suffering and fear of a chronic hepatic condition. The optimistic thoughtlessness of his brother Epimetheus bore bitter fruit, too, as he, suspecting no evil, released diseases from the box of the beautiful Pandora, thereby multiplying the ailments of the world. Tantalus became enmeshed in a more oral fate. For stealing nectar and ambrosia from the table of the gods, he was punished with unquenchable thirst, a condition shared with diabetics. The mythological, where pathology manifests itself as something moralistic/theological, also appears less exalted in legends where the sick, during their lifetimes or posthumously, wander about 'damaged,' emitting uncanny cries or dragging chains through the night with the awkwardness of cripples.

While aetiology is dealt with under the aspect of divine punishment, religious and mythical traditions also carry the belief that prevention and therapy can occur if man, before or after the fact, assumes the possible punishment as penance and atonement. In penance and atonement, we encounter not only the principle of *contraria contrariis* but also that of *similis simile curatur*. Not only must disease be treated with opposites but also with sames. Correspondingly, we expose ourselves prematurely to suffering in order that suffering will leave us in peace. We torment and humiliate ourselves, tending toward suffering as a form of prevention. We drag heavy crosses in supplicational processions, bending our backs under the weight and demonstrating thereby the psychosomatic knowledge that all human hubris is met with buckling, hunchbacked deformities and other manifold vertebral conditions. To prevent a reoccurrence of the epidemic St. Vitus's dance, the populace of Echternach in Luxembourg held annual, chorea-form processions in which participants leaped as if afflicted with the disease. In Babylon, a steer was slaughtered each year in conjunction with the cult of Mithras as if to prevent, by means of this sacrifice of power, the exhaustion of human powers. Similarly, the Aztecs fed their increasingly anemic sun god with the blood and hearts of warriors. Finally, contemporary man seems to attempt to forestall rheumatic chastisement of undue mobility and flexibility by wearing heavy and binding rings and bracelets. Even the discovery of active immunization was preceded in many areas by synonymous cultic practices.

*

Compared with the surgeon who derives his professional designation from the Greek *cheir* 'hand' and who operates, in his blood-spattered cloak, with this and that instrument or with the general practitioner who palpates his patients, examines them, and subjects them to batteries of tests, verbal therapy seems extraordinarily passive. Words are the principal tools, and the hands are restricted to occasional gestures while even advice is given sparingly if at all.

This passivity appears to belong to a special and particular form of service. It requires unusual training to avoid resorting to concrete action or activity of any sort but to withhold emotional energies to the point that they work invisibly behind the scenes.

Verbal therapy includes reflection on and consideration of the disease syndromes that the patient brings. It is not a therapy that assesses on the ground of sensory impressions but one that seeks out the essence, the essential, a process in which sensory impressions play a secondary role. Reflection is actually hermeneutic, the art of phenomenological interpretation—as easy as it is difficult. It seems to be the simplest thing in the world and at the same time the most complex. Reflection would seem to have to recognize the apparently superficial riddle of the Sphinx, the disease syndromes as a general philosopheme. Knowing that recessive character traits somaticize in disease, reflection's task is to extract from the data what is 'wrong' with the patient.

When a young woman is bothered by the continual inflammation of a vaginal infection evoked, for example, by trichomonas, there may be something obstinate present that 'flares up' at attempts to delve into and influence the condition. As a result, the chronic nature of the disorder is effected despite the patient's desire to be helpful and to provide pertinent data concerning her condition. Understanding disease leads us into the realm of impotence and the maddeningly bedeviling.

The moment of successful reflection is often sudden in its effect, yet how it works remains a riddle. Reflection appears to remain efficient even when no further explanation follows, as if the moment of reflection (and it is usually a matter of *a* moment!) developed a psychological effect. It is as if 'telekinesis' were being practiced and all subsequent discussion were but a caring for an already viable embryo. It seems that the occurrence, the 'moment,' lifted disease out of an isolation into which it, in principle, would have had to fall through objective treatment, through 'proper' activity. Re-flection in this sense dilutes, re-lieves, and transforms the density, heaviness, of a disease. It sublimates, re-deems, brings resurrection and, inasmuch as this process is recognized as an essential trait, re-connects the patient with that which was lost and brings him 'together.'

Usually the question "What do I do now?" follows successful reflection. The question is fundamentally false and superfluous. *Recognition was the doing*, and what was most important has already taken place. What now follows will be but a deepening and broadening of what has been recognized. The recognition, the reflection, the comprehension of the essence are the therapy! The recognition changes and motivates us to forms of action that we previously could not or would not have thought of. It is as if thought/spirit and deed/action behaved complementarily, as if they could not be dealt with simultaneously but only sequentially, otherwise excluding one another. And while the effect of spirit develops that much more intensely the more 'paralyzed' therapeutic activity is, the success of activity depends on the motivation of the spirit.

Verbal therapy, therefore, presupposes, requires even, a certain alienation from reality. Too much factual knowledge seems only to lead to ineffectiveness. The greater the number of facts, the greater the danger that essence will fail to emerge, remaining incomprehensible in the factual flood. Verbal therapy in archetypal medicine lives on a limited amount of data. There are certain prerequisites for the application of such data, prerequisites to be found in certain therapists—much as in certain fortune-tellers and faith healers.

*

Language is a psychosomaticum *par excellence.* Language is hybrid in nature, extending from the painless spiritual/subtle, on one hand, to the difficulties and sensuality of the body on the other. Occasionally, it seems possible to build entire worlds with just language, worlds separate from everything else where words are moved back and forth and joined to each other. Appearances deceive, however. Language, too, is so extensively contaminated with the dirt of the earth and by the lust of being that we must fundamentally question whether we can ever lift ourselves above the earth's surface. It seems that we are left little choice but to continue to emit inarticulate cries essentially no different than the cries of apes, the soughs of forest trees, the thunder of falling rocks, the murmuring of a brook, or the rustling of wind in the underbrush.

Actually, speech remains organismic, a twitter. Applied therapeutically, it aligns itself with all methods of psychosomatic treatment which create awareness of our diseased organs, thereby uniting sound and resonance.* Its use belongs as a matter of course to methods of therapy such as Eutonia, Bioenergetics, Feldendreis Training, etc., those methods which intensify awareness of the body and for the body's ailing as well, so that the latter has no choice but to change. Speech by itself has the same effect when sufficiently laden with physical and sensual sensations of the respective disease. Speech should, in this context, not be too abstract; its terminology should derive neither from empirical science nor from quasi-pure philosophy. Speech should lead into spirit and thereby make sublime that of which it speaks. At the same time, it should remain imaginal,

* The Indo-Germanic root of speech is *pers* which means 'resonance.' Speech in this sense becomes, so to speak, the resounding of physical existence.

directed toward primal images, toward archetypal images where content and form become identical. Dialogue during a therapeutic hour is a multifaceted reality in which, as we know, the seating order, the positional attitudes of therapist and patient, the melody of what is said or spoken, the gestures, etc., all have their place and worth. The dialogue is a complex interaction, the discussion being actually a mutual touching. It comes close to being physical, and to that extent it is also treatment, a laying-on of hands. The patient also evidences all those reactions which a patient under other, more concrete treatment might demonstrate: he winces or manifests other signs of pain; he imagines that he is being scrutinized and twists and turns because of the probing examination. He might suddenly register a chill or feel relieved when it is over, or it may seem to him as if he had been salved with cooling balsam. After the therapy hour, he may feel restored and comforted or exhausted. In other words, manipulation and handling occur as much in the analytical consulting room as they do on the surgeon's examining table. If now and again the opinion is expressed that analytical consultations are no more intense than a tea party, we ought not to forget that visits to the doctor are themselves often nothing more than *kaffee klatsch*.

We often assume, somewhat erroneously, that the predecessors of practitioners of verbal therapy are to be found especially among priests. In making this assumption, we probably have in mind the notion that physical contact is of secondary importance in both forms of relationship. Following what has been said above, this notion carries only limited validity. The predecessors of verbal therapists are rather all those who, in one form or another, practice the art of healing. This applies as much to faith healers as to those who have incised, cauterized, or medicated. If we concede any power to therapeutic language, that power derives its effectiveness from the hybrid capacity of language to be both physical and spiritual reality.

*

Since empirical medicine thinks in terms of open systems, it has had to develop a particularly serious ethic. For empirical medicine, facts are and remain unique, while disease and health carry the stamp of unquestionable reality. They are non-interchangeable and, as such, arise causally. Whatever is takes on a leaden reality and becomes something which must be talked about. In empirical medicine and in an era dominated by its perspective, the flood of information must of necessity snowball: education becomes a life or death matter. Because facts are so unique (with certain temporal limitations due to change), they must be accorded the highest seriousness.

Empirical medicine also holds to the conception of life as a linear process in which any 'after' cannot be a 'before.' This tenet places empirical medicine in the position of having to hold the brow unflinchingly wrinkled and the eyebrows perpetually and meaningfully raised. The image of life as a linear process extending from health to disease and from there to death (according to which "health" means 'life') compels empirical medicine to become emergency medicine, and the overall development tends to make intensive care units out of entire countries.

While the ethic of empirical medicine is one of serious morality, such does not apply to archetypal medicine. Since archetypal medicine thinks in closed systems wherein elements are arranged in polarities and derive value only in relation to something else, a more a-moral ethic results. In principle nothing is unique. For that matter, what appeared unique at one point may shortly revert to just the opposite. Consequently, information is no longer decisive, for over all information hangs the specter of futility and uselessness. Events, even those of medical significance, take on something of Goethe's "Gestaltung, Umgestaltung, des ewigen Sinnes ewige Unterhaltung" ("Formation, transformation, of meaning eternal, eternal diversion").

When we consider, in addition to the differences in ethics, that archetypal medicine employs facts primarily as the starting point for intuiting essence (for example, discussion of a case of anemia shifts to considerations of things pale, washed-out, and white), the diversionary quality of medical reality is further increased. It is as if for archetypal medicine everything were but half-real, as if a final smile or laugh never disappeared, and that a constant incredulity remained that Nature really intended to be so serious with us. It is as if our human world carried the quality of a fata morgana, easily confused with meaninglessness. Where intuition is practiced, reality always retains the quality of sorcery and, therefore, the ethic of archetypal medicine tends toward *irony*. Despite all existentialism, life still retains something virtual.

If the object of empirical medicine is a serious matter, then the doctor who deals with it must himself be serious. Usually he is revered, revered with the same reverence as was the due of the Greek god Apollo, who, as a marble-white, exalted figure of anatomical perfection, looked out over the Gulf of Corinth from the heights of Delphi. As the progenitor of all doctors, Apollo conquered Python, a snake representing everything disgusting, misanthropic, malignant, and disease- and death-dealing. Apollo was a victor, a conqueror, a sun god, qualities retained by his medical descendants. But this noble heritage can undermine itself. It seems as if the irony referred to above were compelled to proliferate wildly as outraged cynicism when not accorded its rightful place in the scheme of things.

Archetypal medicine pays homage to Apollo's brother, Mercury or Hermes, a god far less symmetrical and healthy. Mercury sees to it that everything is connected to everything else, so that the cosmos remains a closed system. He practices magic and possesses wit, something that cannot be said for Apollo. His smile is archaic. While the Apollonian has remained dominant, its characteristics preserved through the centuries by a Christian, light-above-and-dark-below world, Mercury has led more of an apocryphal, secret existence. He finds reverence among subcultures, among those, for instance, that fall under the heading of alchemy. So it is even today.

It belongs to the nature of the Apollonian that man feels compelled to regard his own existence—and being in general—as miraculous. It is as if man were implanted with a fundamental conviction, thanks to which everything is capable of appearing good. This primary belief becomes suspect when, unquestioned, it turns into a mania as is the case today. Whenever the sun darkens, victims, particularly heart victims, are sacrificed as they were at the time of the Aztecs. The economic value of the religion of miraculous existence is incontestable: it creates innumerable jobs and consumes enormous amounts of energy.

What applies to our era as a whole applies to empirical medicine specifically. For empirical medicine, a sick patient is essentially a *privatio boni*, a lessened, misshapen Good, the pillaging of something regarded as a legitimate wholeness. Like our entire era, empirical medicine has its specific heroic task in restoring what is missing, a task it unswervingly pursues despite the similarities to Sisyphus's task. Empirical medicine's attitude includes an a priori celebration of—a jubilation to—creation, while everything which does not correspond to creation separates out as mistake and error.

Archetypal medicine does not share this attitude. Serving a mercurial god possessing numerous connections to death and dying, archetypal medicine's ethic does not draw its sustenance from an unquestioned celebration. Its hermetic characteristics enable archetypal medicine from the outset to experience all being—and correspondingly, not least of all, human existence—as a necessary evil. Just as we can assume that flowers are what *really* matters and that compost merely serves to further blooming or that rotting and spoilage are but an inevitable disappointment, so can we also regard the compost itself as primary, that from which wonders sprout. While a position of primary jubilation must needs be supported with all sorts of persistence, tricks, lies, etc., so that its volume does not diminish, archetypal medicine experiences many things as the result of grace.

In contrast with empirical medicine which, consciously or unconsciously, reveres all life and therewith human existence, archetypal medicine resounds with *derision*. There reigns a blaspheming and a narcissistic aggrievedness. In archetypal medicine, neither illness nor death is an error of Nature but rather an apparently unavoidable, quasi-criminal negligence. If our form of life, a hybrid of desire and torment, was all that Nature could allow to proliferate from the inorganic, Nature could just as well have left well enough alone. Consequently, archetypal medicine is somewhat vengeful, is allied with the Devil, and risks his fate. We could designate such an ethical fundament as morbid or morbistic. *Morbism*, correspondingly, would be the theory that all life, particularly human life, exists only as disease or as health in conjunction with disease. In no wise is this theory new: it resonates with medieval and romantic tones, audible to a kind of individual characterized logically as *morbidezza*.

*

To promote a better understanding of what archetypal medicine could be, it has been portrayed as if we were dealing with something clear-cut, something distinct in everyday practice from empirical medicine. The impression is misleading. Neither can the two forms of medicine be completely separated nor are there any doctors that practice exclusively one or the other. In reality, the difference is much more a question of respective tendencies in which there is the widest variation.

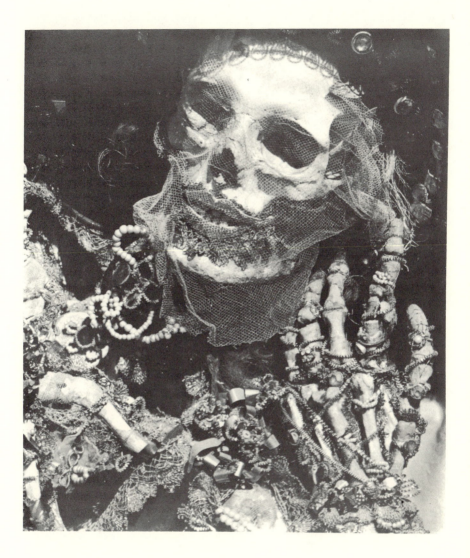

Baroque relics of St. Felix. The worship of the bones of martyrs is not only of religious import but is related to the medical theory according to which similars are treated with similars, *similis simile.*

Praxis

Natura *naturat*: Nature experiences and perceives herself, and without her nothing is that is. Her experience and perception follow certain fundamental patterns or *archetypes*. Through the archetypes, everything is related to everything else and demonstrates common characteristics, analogies, and kinships. Another way of stating the same phenomenon is as the "Sympathy of All Things." This kinship or relationship also exists among disease syndromes so that, for example, anemia might be seen to correspond to the early-morning rays of the sun which the Aztecs perceived as being weak, cold, and pale.

The kinship among disease syndromes, though, is primarily a question of perception: our sense of reality usually registers in terms of differences, not of similarities. Similarity or kinship, however, is more substantial or 'essential' than differences, similarity being bound to intuition and to a sense of essence. The kinship of diseases winds through all existence and, correspondingly, can be enriched, amplified, and evolved from myths, philosophies, and folklore medicine which, from earliest times, has served mankind as a way of understanding all that befell him. These patterns are not merely intellectual or spiritual perceptions of man's destiny but can be taken quite literally and can apply to medicine as well. Amplification is therefore a continual expansion of possibilities of experience, goes hand-in-hand with changes in our physical being, and is capable of 'diluting' or 'sublimating' such changes in the sense of therapeutic effects. This is why the discussion in the following chapter on asthmatic constriction refers to bedeviling spirits, nightmares, and invincible mountain gods—not simply as demonstrations of armchair erudition, but because the experience of the disease itself resonates through them. Were these considerations but knowledge devoid of any experiential referent, they would not only lack any therapeutic effect, but also any resulting diagnosis would want for the seasoning of medical knowledge.

Only because we can perceive existence in an analogically structured fashion—and because of the potential or actual relationship among diseases—is it possible to practice medicine in the first place. The relationship between the one who treats and the one who is treated, and vice versa, is given a priori. An understanding attitude toward the patient is primary. The doctor, the one who treats, complements the relationship to the patient with his experience and knowledge. His knowledge is based principally on *theoria*, not merely an objective, detached knowing, but the knowing of 'experiencing with.' The theoretical attitude is fundamentally one of embodying; diagnosis is not a seeing through, but a living through; and therapy itself draws from a participation in a cult-like bond. In archetypal medicine, everything—and everyone—joins in and contributes to the discussion.

Our theme, then (by no means a new one!), is one of a theory of perception. If, as Goethe says, the eye sees the sun because it (the eye) has sun-like qualities, then one should also say that man perceives illness because he himself is ill and can *be* ill! There is a morbid kinship with everything that allows us to perceive morbidity. If words alone can have a therapeutic value, they do so only insofar as they evoke a corporeal sense of this morbid relationship.

*

The practical section is arranged according to specific diseases and their syndromes, not according to empirical medicine's perspective of diseases as self-contained units. In empirical medicine, general pathology takes precedence over specific pathology. The selected syndromes which follow have been taken from various medical disciplines. Other syndromes, though, could just as well have been chosen: spasmodic conditions or angina pectoris, edema or headaches, gallstones, diarrhea, or senility would have been equally suited as examples for the concepts of archetypal medicine.

The individual chapters are complete in themselves and, depending on the syndromes, place varying emphasis on genetic, aetiological, pathogenetic, and therapeutic aspects. Consideration of the question of locus, where a particular disease originates, is superfluous in archetypal medicine. The diseased part of the anatomy plays less the role of the focused effects of environmental conflicts and more the role of that environmental component in which fate or destiny finds its fulfillment. Necessary references to anatomy, physiology, and pathology are provided since overall understanding of the concepts depends upon a clearly defined point of departure. Usually such existing knowledge finds a place in psychosomatic literature. Always, though, the unity of the theory of archetypal medicine has priority: what is a priori in medical knowledge precedes that which is a posteriori.

Asthmatic Constriction

THE characteristic constriction we call asthma is mainly a disease syndrome which expresses itself to varying degrees in our bodies. On the one hand, there may be no appreciable physical effect, while on the other it may irrevocably lead to death. Bronchial asthma is one of the best known forms of the disorder—probably because of its unpredictable attacks. Although the attacks are the most spectacular aspect of bronchial asthma, the intervening intervals are not nearly as dramatic. Like most diseases of particular importance to man, asthma is episodic in nature, resulting in an increasing degree of invalidism. This pattern corresponds to a general pattern in living beings which, like a cascade, brings death inexorably, step-by-step, closer.

We experience an asthma attack as suffocation, threatening our very lives. It is as if the bronchial passages were suddenly seized by panic and the dominant need of the lungs below (usually taken for granted!) were ignored. The process of exhaling, in particular, is affected or choked off. The patient braces himself in order to keep the air passages as open as possible, even as fear registers in his eyes. His face discolors, taking on a bluish tinge. His breath comes in rasps and whistles. Toward the end of the attack, the patient coughs and expectorates. The overall effect is of someone who has been startled by something terrible and unknown and who has fixed his attention on it. Not infrequently, the attacks take place when they are least expected. Conspicuous is the characteristic incongruity between the sensational quality of the attack and the relative composure with which the patient answers questions posed to him. His voice can sound surprisingly disinterested, his thinking clear and logical. It is as if the patient sought to maintain his self-control to the last breath with no consideration of the apocalyptic event he has been caught in.

An internist would tell us that bronchial asthma results from spasms in certain parts of the bronchi, from inflammation and swelling of the bronchial mucous membranes, and from an accumulation of phlegm in the upper air passages. The inhaled air is blocked as a result, a phenomenon which in time causes the lungs to contract of their own accord, creating cavities. These cavities are referred to as emphysema. The most severe injury is caused by the so-called "asthmatic status," an attack which can continue unabated for days at a time. For the patient, asthmatic status is a special torment. It often ends in death since the pressure in the lungs can become so severe that it impedes the supply of blood to the lungs. Because of the resistance in the lungs, the right side of the heart has to work harder, frequently decompensating to the point of death.

Even though a patient does die from a bronchial attack, the pathologist may not discover any noticeable changes at the postmortem. Bronchial asthma is like many other human ailments inasmuch as a patient can die from the disorder even when the degree of somatization is relatively low. Exceptionally, there may be no posthumous findings of pathology. A sudden death of this kind corresponds directly to what ethnologists call a "voodoo death," as when a tribesman dies unexpectedly after having received a threatening visitation. An acute, sudden death from bronchial asthma is but a specialized form of the same thing. Actually, most forms of human death can be regarded as "voodoo deaths," since the same processes are always involved—the only difference is that the patient dies sometimes after the first such visitation, sometimes only after a number of visitations. The principle holds true not only for death from a bronchial attack but also for death from an infarct or an apoplectic seizure as well. Even the first attacks of bronchial asthma can be lethal, although death usually plays according to set rules and generally occurs only after that patient has developed a history of bronchial disorders.

*

Bronchial asthma is the pulmonary somatization of a missed opportunity for silence and the feeling of meaningless insignificance. Consequently, the disorder will especially afflict those who are partially or completely unaware of their compulsive need to dominate others, who consider their attitude toward life 'inspired,' and who 'catch their breath' when someone other than themselves has the last word. When exhalation is blocked, their speech, as well as their breath, is 'taken away.' Asthmatics are said to have a tendency to be idealistic and ethically pretentious. This can go so far that they become tyrants for whom the slightest contradiction is interpreted as a frontal attack upon their right to exist. Since any attempt to correct their arrogance is experienced as a blow, they often consolidate their idealism in a formal structure to insure their security. Although they may well manage to achieve their goals in their relationships with others, their susceptibility and vulnerability to the treacherous attacks of their condition only increase. The more their ideals of simplicity, purity, and clarity are achieved and maintained by dominating themselves and others, the greater the likelihood of an attack of their inner disorder and the greater their hyper-sensitivity.

The disorder is by no means selective in its choice of triggering agents. The patient's hyper-sensitivity seeks out noxae, even among the most unexpected things. While asthma is considered an allergic disease, particular environmental factors have little importance in the outbreak of an attack. A specific allergen can be shown to be involved in only twenty percent of asthma cases. Even where a specific allergen *is* involved, patients may suffer attacks in the absence of that allergen. In addition, not only con-crete allergic agents in the form of house dust, pollen, and pet hair trigger attacks but *pictures* of animals, plants, smoking locomotives, and the like as well. Sometimes even the sight of a high mountain or another person who is perceived as being somehow superior, 'above,' the patient will bring on an attack. It seems as if anything which threatens the asthmatic's 'inspired' way of life or attitude is sufficient to internally choke or smother him.

The general irrelevance of triggering agents is something that asthma, bronchial asthma, has in common with numerous other human diseases. On the basis of experience, almost *all diseases would have to be classified as allergies*, because they all seek their noxae out of a kind of hyper-sensitivity, making what is otherwise harmless into disease-evoking elements.

*

The insight and psychological understanding we have for the asthmatic process directly contradict the occasional contention that asthma results from a familial or pedagogic milieu. Actu-ally, inheritance or an inherited disposition seems to play a preponderant role as demonstrated by research done with twins. The incidence of asthma among monozygotic twins is twice as great as that among bi-zygotic twins, indicating that the environmental factors are of less importance than inheritance. There seems to exist a predisposition for the disorder in 'asthmatic families' which determines their lifestyle and stand-ards for success. The same predisposition effects the appropriate somatization, fulfilling thereby Nature's task of disintegration and 'dis-posing.'

Even in early childhood the predisposition has harnessed the environment to its purposes, seeing to it that parents and teachers are forced into behavioral patterns which will con-tribute to the formation of the 'asthmatic' personality. From the beginning, the paradox of dominance on the one hand and pettiness on the other locates in the respiratory system causing behavior which particularly taxes the patience of the mother. Patients' mothers are unjustly viewed as causal factors in the aetiology of the disorder.

The confusion of motherly feelings toward the child finds expression in the mother's attempts to spoil the poor little dear. She tends to his needs with obtrusive tenderness and an abundance of physical closeness and warmth. She actually 'smothers' him with warmth and food. At the same time, though, she defends herself against her child's demands and harbors hostile feelings or apathy toward him. The end result is a completely confused relationship between mother and child. While the mother is torn between feelings of loving concern and hate, the child's feelings vary from authoritative demands to powerlessness. The pattern established and experienced in the nursery is repeated in later life, although the later experiences should not be attributed any particular causal significance. The asthmatic's mood swings from a sense of the apocalyptic to ethereal highs of all kinds. Accordingly, he later manipulates friends and husband or wife in the same manner he did parents and teachers. The more he is able to maintain a position of dominance, the more assuredly will he suffer from collapses.

*

The pattern just described finds expression in pathognomonic dreams—dreams from which the patient awakens with symptoms characteristic to his condition. The dream and the syndrome are closely related and provide reciprocal amplification and interpretation. The following dream is such a pathognomonic one, dreamt by a forty-one-year-old man who, at the time, was an assistant professor of Tibetan studies. He awoke from the dream with an asthmatic attack.

In Vienna, on the Praterstern, I am suspected of having committed murder, since everywhere I have been seen bodies have been discovered. I suggest to the police that from now on they accompany me and guard me day and night. This way they will soon be able to determine that I have nothing to do with these deaths. The police get in their car and follow me. Suddenly the earth begins to tremble as if there were an earthquake or a landslide. Dust and dirt swirl in the air. I sink deeper and deeper. Earth begins to cover me. I scream for my grandparents. At the end of the dream I am hurrying naked from one square to another while chunks of earth fall off of me.

The patient was an aspiring man who sought in Tibetan philosophy the spiritual purity which would make the worries in his life bearable. He was always studiously polite, even submissive. He loved spirited, intellectual conversations and was imbued with the necessity of personal integrity. He always carried a large briefcase with him where all sorts of books as well as publications which he himself had written could be found. His clothes were usually grimy, and he gave the impression of needing a bath and of having let himself go to seed.

The dream signifies that, at that point in time when the patient demanded definitive proof of his impeccable integrity, catastrophe broke in upon him. It would appear that this were the demand which set the whole chain of events in motion. He wanted to have nothing to do with suspicions, with evil or antisocial elements, and therefore selected the most stringent means of proof.

His downfall is massive in its proportions, the air practically unbreathable and filled with dirt, stones, and clouds of dust. The dream has translated the patient's physical process into an apocalypse, delivering point for point a transposition of psychic and physical events into the language of images and thence to comprehension. The dream is, therefore, "pathognomonic"— characteristic of the disease, in other words.

*

A majority of asthmatic attacks and asthma-like conditions occur during sleep—usually during phases of emotional dreaming, or REM phases. These dreams are often similar to reports from German folklore concerning encounters with a creature called an "alp," the bringer of nightmares. According to legend, the alp slipped through a crack under the door or through a keyhole, down the chimney or other furtive passage into the bedroom. At most there would be a sound like the scuttling of mice or the light footfall of a cat. Suddenly the alp would leap in a single bound onto the bed and slowly crawl upward, from the dreamer's feet to his chest, weighing him down with its weight. It would squeeze the dreamer's throat, steal his breath away, or stick its finger or its hairy tongue into the dreamer's mouth. Such occurrences happened also to children who would whimper or awaken in shock.

Asthmatic "alp" dreams or nightmares point to the subtle way the disorder may begin, as if on the light tread of a cat's paws. When patients are questioned in detail about their dreams, the generalized pattern of classical alp dreams begins to emerge. It is not rare for these dreams to transpose physical sensations into highly grotesque images, a fact which would support the assumption that the legendary traditions are based on actual perceptions and not upon someone's mere fantasy. In other words, it is completely possible for an asthma patient to have the feeling that something which corresponds to an alp is sitting on his chest or wrenching his mouth open as if to count his teeth, blowing its breath down his throat.

After what has been said about the asthmatic and his relationship to the mother, it is not surprising that the legendary alp corresponds to the asthmatic's experience of 'mother' as a threatening, overwhelming mass. The alp often appears in feminine form, as a white woman, for instance, or as an old crone with a long nose, bulging eyes, ice-cold hands, long, stringy hair, and wide, shuffling pentagonal or toadlike feet. More often, though, it is amorphous, ugly, repulsively moist, has a large head and long, pendulous breasts like cow udders, or it takes shape as a fog or a draft. Hair figures significantly in the appearance of the alp, especially when it assumes forms other than furry animals. One of its preferred animal forms is that of the martin, a creature whose name is said to be related to the German *Mahr* 'tale,' *Maerchen* 'fairytale,' and to the English "mare" in "nightmare." The alp may even select smoke as its avatar as in Switzerland where it is called *Toggeli*, a name which also applies to the alp as a cat. Finally, the alp may assume the shape or guise of objects in the bedroom itself: straw or corn cobs from mattresses, woolen yarn or thread, and human hair. Does not the wide variety of shapes in which the alp appears remind us of the innumerable harmful agents which allergists have blamed as the cause or source of asthma? Does it not occur to the observer that the intrigues of these various forms have something to do with the basic personality of the asthmatic and with his earlier, childhood experiences?

By nature, the alp is related to the witch in her significance as a kind of uncanny mother-figure. Like the witch, the alp is carried or borne by the wind, and just as the witch sends disease as the stabbing pain of her spells, the alp strikes its victims with "belemnite" or "thunder stone." Its deeds are regarded less as being intentionally evil and rather more as clumsiness and oafishness. In like manner, we have to view the behavior of "asthmatic mothers" not as wickedness as much as an undifferentiated motherliness that crushes children to death out of sheer love. It is much more motherly primitivity than perfidy which complements the predisposition of the child.

*

Asthmatics' inflated lifestyle combines with an expiratory hostility usually vented in explosive staccatos. Asthmatics, themselves, are aware of the hostility. Often they would just as soon that the whole world would blow up and disintegrate. A primal scream would be their preferred mode of expression. Yet, even the slightest fantasy or thought of animosity gets stuck, so to speak, in their lungs. Anything which issues from a body opening can bode ill, and usually the best the asthmatic can manage is a cough or some discharge. Everything that issues from the body, everything that begins with "ex," can be inherently malevolent, whether it be exanthema, skin exudations, or asthmatic expectorate which forms as a vitreous, viscous mucous in the constricted bronchi, contributing to the blockage of expiration. Coughing and discharge are expressions of a declaration of intention which should properly take a more differentiated form such as screaming curses or orders.

As part of the inhalation therapy which asthmatics undergo, the attempt is made to isolate these primitive forms of expression and to develop them into higher, more human communication. Inhalation therapy converts aggressiveness into the ex-pression of formal speech patterns, a revised version of a method used by folk medicine hundreds of years ago to enable asthmatics to escape the stranglehold of the alp. In those days, asthmatics had to beat out the form of a cross three times on their gums with their tongues, let out a curse or a scream, pray at the top of their lungs, or shout out the name of the repulsive alp itself. These procedures were accompanied by jerking motions with the entire body and the following words: "Adiuto te, satanae diabolus, aelfae . . . ut refugiatur ab homine illo" ("I banish you, Satan, alp; be gone from this person!").

*

It is well-known that bronchial asthma responds especially well to high altitudes: asthma in children at one time was even treated with flights in airplanes. Scientists managed to come up with numerous physical and chemical explanations for the phenomenon but, as is frequently the case, none of the explanations worked out. Rather, they remain scanty and contested hypotheses which, compared with contributions from poetry, myth, and religion concerning heights and exaltation, seem rather deficient in their thought content, no matter how much intellectual ability and energy have gone into them.

We can understand that the asthmatic, moving through life with the nightmare of the alp's oppression lurking in his lungs, experiences the elevation of mountainous regions as a salvation. In the higher altitudes, the asthmatic's inspirational lifestyle and the heroism related to it, his love of the pure, the clear, and of the order of the intellect, find their place. In the mountains, the light is often lovely and clear, the air is subtly pure and cool, and the panoramas open into distance as well as depth. All these qualities are characteristic of a place where the asthmatic could live free from the fear of his condition.

What takes place at higher elevations can also be effected by certain drugs: those, for instance, that result in a feeling of euphoria. Corticoids, the hormones produced by the cortex of the suprarenal gland, serve not only to reduce the swelling of the mucous lining of the bronchi but also to engender a psychic state characterized by a feeling of happiness due to some unspecific hormonal effect. The hormone produced by the adrenal medulla, adrenalin, and its derivatives have a similar effect: not only do they relax the tonus of the flat musculature of the bronchi, they also serve to stimulate the entire organism, thereby evoking a feeling of great freedom.

High altitudes, then, like the medication prescribed for asthmatic therapy, bring about a fundamental biological transformation in the patient, a condition which directly precedes aeroembolism or mountain sickness (caisson disease) of low-grade stimulation usually of a pleasant or euphoric nature. The asthmatic feels good, the air is fresh, climbing is easy and effortless, and he could go on for hours. Everyday worries fall by the wayside, yielding to a carefree mood and heightened awareness of everything in sight. The climber revels in movement. Like the resonating tones of the alp-horn, exhalation comes as a blessing from the otherwise oppressive alp, a super-elevation of release. Occasionally, the climber's mood changes abruptly into irritation, impetuosity, or anxiety, being most affected by the peaks, ridges, and plateaus, by those over-towering, surpassing parts of the landscape. It is as if the patient had fallen into the hands of the mountain gods, as much a part of the experience of higher elevations as the long rays of the sun and the blue and white colors of the landscape. It is here that a sunrise takes on qualities of the numinous, becomes revelation and enlightenment all in one, where contrasts between light and dark achieve a particular pregnancy, contributing to the sensation of clear and distinct order. It is understandable that convents and monasteries have been built here and there in the mountains so that the members of the various religious orders can live in proximity to that ethereal light which spreads its rays across the world each morning.

Not only does the light take on ethereal properties in the mountains, but so do the winds; one is tempted to say the breezes as well. There breezes are not only free of mist and fog but—more decisive for the asthmatic—also of dust and pollen particles. The air is often aromatic, resinous or, at the very least, lacking the odorous pollutants so common at lower elevations. Finally, the sensation of vast expanses is enough to bring anyone around as the view extends into seemingly bottomless depths or out to the farthest valley. The world takes on vertical qualities here, imbued with the aesthetic and completely alien to the driven human compulsiveness below. Life in the mountains is hardly livable, and the prospect of a bleak, rocky, unproductive existence absolves the asthmatic sufferer of the duty to "go forth and multiply."

The sense of the religious which appears at higher elevations belongs to the "mountain-top experiences" of rapture and divine voices. Yet not only does the Christian God speak from the aura of dawn, but also above the shimmering white of the eternal snows shine gods of many other religions, not the least of whom is Saturn, enthroned in alchemy on the mountain. Lord of unchanging, non-chronological time, Saturn is a god of a cold and dry nature connected to the rocks and crags in his immutability. As Cronos/Saturn, he is the spirit of original order in its irrefutable and irrevocable state.

The physical, medical methods of treatment for bronchial asthma are actually quite effective and exemplify in general the treatment principle of modern medicine: *contraria contrariis*. The drugs employed all fall into the category of "anti," like *anti*asthmatic corticoids, *anti*biotics, and *anti*allergics. In point of fact, this principle promotes a return to the state of health which gave rise to the disease, a return to the very source of the disorder! In psychoanalytic terms we would say that the treatment promotes "resistance," but inasmuch as it strengthens resistance, it serves to perpetuate the pathognomonic pattern. While the asthmatic undoubtedly returns to a state of symptom-free euphoria with medicinal sleights-of-hand, at the same time the demons which plagued him are reconstellated. Somatic treatment of bronchial asthma predominates in medical treatment; its effect lies in creating health in an uncritical manner and therewith the precondition for the illness it heals. Medical treatment, in other words, is capable of opening the way for an increase in inappropriate attitudes and Apollonian illusions. Although a blessing, it is still a curse.

When asthma is treated unquestioningly through the removal of symptoms, experience shows that we can count on considerably more relapses and complications than when respect is given to the disease. As we know, the disease has a point to make! A verbal, psychotherapeutic approach not only questions the value of the asthmatic's attempts to escape from his imaginary persecutors (such attempts being of a Sisyphus nature anyway) but also encourages a reevaluation of everything considered to be immature, negative, and inferior which plagues the patient as nightmares. The immature, negative, and inferior aspects normally smothered by the alp do not lack in value but are meaningful psychic conditions which, for example, enable us to pass more 'invisibly' through life. In addition to the reevaluation, it is also essential that the patient be led to the insight that not only the 'outer' world is peopled with alps or allergens but also the 'inner' world of every individual.

The therapeutic approach of archetypal medicine, without renouncing the practices of modern, somatic techniques, revolves around a *tertium*, a third between the somatic and the psychic, catering to one without ignoring the other. Archetypal medicine would treat asthma on the basis of "either *and* or" (as opposed to "either/or") and is reminiscent of the fairytale of "The Spirit in the Bottle." As the story goes, a wanderer discovered a glass bottle containing a very agitated being demanding to be set free. No sooner was he out of the bottle than he turned into a terrible goblin intent upon murdering his deliverer, freedom having induced wantonness. Using a trick, the wanderer persuaded the spirit to return to this original abode, and the discussion about setting him free continued until a compromise acceptable to both was reached. This kind of compromise is the position of the third which perceives humility in the most peremptory expression or perceives the repressiveness (as well as the legitimacy) of a sense of our own smallness.

tive form, histamine is found in various human organs such as the histiocytes of the blood, in the lungs, and in the skin. When activated, it dilates arterioles and capillaries, the smallest extensions of the arterial system, increasing their permeability and allowing serous fluid to pass into the surrounding areas, a process which may result in edema. (In addition to the effects of histamine, there is also the factor of the excitation of the nerve endings.) The determining role of histamine for *pruritus* is deduced from the observation that antihistamines provide immediate relief from the symptoms. It is not surprising that antihistamines also have an ataractic or tranquilizing effect: chemically they were the first substances used in psychiatry which offered effective relief from psychotic anxieties of imaginary persecution and torment. Antihistamines belong to the group of compounds which can protect us from falling prey to the consuming fires of some chance passion or affect.

Itching is the somatic form of a number of erotic, hostile, even spiritual affects occurring particularly when we imagine that we have such affects under control and especially at times when this illusion of control is interrupted by a sudden and unexpected state of isolation. This holds true for numerous pruriginous skin conditions accompanied to a greater or lesser degree by physical symptoms. This seems to be the case for psoriasis which tends to pop up in moments when a prudish attitude of non-involvement is confronted in unusual ways by gregarious drives. It is also the case for allergic eczema whose pointed, itching, dermal granulations manifest themselves at times when a state of "anergy," an absence of emotional reaction, is contrasted by pronounced impulses for revenge or self-preservation. Children as well as adults are affected by these conditions. Milk allergy, an evolutionary precursor of eczema, is a child's way of defending itself against an overly 'ascetic' mother and the threat of isolation. Allergic nettle rash, *urticaria*, whose onset can be characterized by a pronounced itching, is a similar condition. It especially tends to occur when we are mired, more or less consciously, in fruitless, ad absurdum complaints against man and nature, when the repressed desire to strike back with 'inflamma-tory' comments is pathologized and appears as an itching 'in-flammation.'

The principle to which I have alluded, that itching in some form or other overcomes us when we have unwittingly settled into a state of "anergic" isolation, should also hold true for certain delusional states. I am talking about cases in which patients are plagued by delusions of dermal parasites and insects to the point of such despair and such a need to scratch that their con-dition must be designated "psychotic." The process is not unlike the outbreak of *pruriginous* sensations with neurotic compulsive patients whose exaggerated sense of hygiene and perfectionism connected with washing and cleanliness rituals drives them insane.

What holds true for other disease syndromes also applies to itching: somatic manifestations adhere to certain *rules of inten-sity*. *Pruritus* can appear as the so-called *pruritus sine materia*, that is, without any significant physical changes. On the other hand, as *pruritus cum materia*, it manifests itself through any one of a number of physical ailments. We are not talking about skin dis-orders per se such as psoriasis, eczema, *urticaria*, or the condi-tions caused by parasites like lice, fleas, and mites. Rather, the reference here is to internal disorders which *pruritus* can, in varying degrees, 'use': liver disorders, diabetes mellitus, chronic kidney conditions, carcinomas of internal organs, enlargement of the prostate, anemia, and so forth. The way the body regis-ters itching is equivalent to other, sometimes similar conditions, making no significant distinction between itching and shiver-ing, twitching, or throbbing. This equivalence is reflected in the tradition of fortunetelling where all of these sensations are attributed a similar mantic importance, signifying something taking place or which would take place outside or beyond the customary field of perception. Itching was not regarded as being of greater mantic significance than any of the other symptoms.

The belief in the mantic implications of *pruritus* is extremely widespread and goes back to early antiquity. In many areas it has resulted in its own literature as was the case for dream interpretation and palmistry. The so-called "Twitch Books" exist in Greek, Hebrew, Turkish, Roumanian, and Slavic versions, and isolated records have been found throughout northern Europe. Apparently, the first to write such a book was Poseidonios, a Stoic with a lively interest in folklore. On the other hand, Cicero in his *De Divinatione* mentions nothing of such practices, considering them to be nothing but superstition and not deserving of serious consideration. The sole Greek version of a "Twitch Book" preserved to the present day carries the name of Melampus, a prophet and priest, as its author.

The Middle Ages accepted the superstitions connected with itching as a vital part of the heritage of antiquity as shown by the polemics of the Christian writers of the time: St. Augustine called them a jumble of totally meaningless observations. The church labeled those who made pronouncements on the future or the unknown on the basis of twitching and itching *salisatores* (*salire* 'to jump,' 'to twitch'), their practices "jumping," and frequently chastised them. "Jumping" is in no wise a thing of the past, certain elements having managed to survive until the present. The best known example is the belief that a change in the weather is indicated when an old scar itches. In Shakespeare's *Macbeth*, one witch says to another, "by the prickling of my thumbs, something wicked this way comes." Occasionally, the twitching of an eyelid will be ascribed a prophetic significance, a sign that a joyful or tragic occurrence, an unexpected visit, perhaps, is in the offing. The other, practically innumerable, meanings attributed to twitches and itches on various parts of the body have not stood the test of time except as part of the "Twitch Books."

Psychosomatic medicine in general and archetypal medicine in particular cannot help but be *mantic*! For archetypal medicine, disease syndromes are the physical manifestation of psychic processes engendered in conjunction with triggering factors in the outer world, something of which we at best are only subliminally conscious. It is, therefore, no wonder that somatic disorders are understood as a signal for the unexpected. We can also understand why a number of pathological phenomena are dealt with both by psychosomatic medicine as well as by folklore prophecy. Further, we can see how the decline of an empire could be deduced from a deformed gall bladder or changes in the liver as the result of a mantic examination of the viscera for the benefit of the reigning king: when gall's bitterness is not released for the good of the country, it leads to sickliness and misery.

*

It is not only during seances that scratching heralds the opening of the spirit world but wherever we find the lowly itch. The etymology of the word "scratch" provides a number of words applicable to the study of *pruritus*, words all having to do with itching and formed from the root *greb* over a period of centuries. In German we find *graben* 'to dig,' as in 'to dig a grave,' and *gruebeln* 'to meditate or ruminate,' a digging up and sorting through. In English there is the word "grave" in all of its implications and variations. We also have creeping, crabbing, and crawling, as well as the German *Krabbe* 'crab,' *Krebs* 'crawfish' or 'cancer,' and *Kraetze* 'scab' or 'scabies.' One has the sense of something buglike, that 'bugs,' bothers, is creepy and, at the same time, bores holes in order to discover something. The application being much wider than simply disorders of the skin: depressive patients, for example, ruminate, brood, go over and over the same material much as do philosophers or researchers. Implied, at least in the constructive meaning of the word, is a 'scratching' or striking of a divine spark, and bringing of insight and evidence from which one is 'fired up' and inspired!

*

Freudian psychoanalysts regard itching as the expression of sexual desires and interpret boring and scratching as masturbatory equivalents. To support this theory, psychoanalysts cite the facts that various languages use the same word for tickling and sexual intercourse, that games and rhymes which 'tickle' the sense of humor have an aphrodisiac effect, or that girls who are especially ticklish become less so when they begin having intercourse on a regular basis. There are even some folklore traditions in which ticklishness is considered a proof of virginity. Scratching frequently provides a very pleasant sensation which explains the term "pruriginous onanism." The so-called *furor eroticus* is a condition in which the patient scratches so uncontrollably that it is considered 'neuropathic' because of its similarity to obsessive nailbiting. In some forms of neuroses, orgasm is induced by the scratching of certain skin areas. This is given as justification for not prescribing carbonic acid baths for patients whose skin is highly erogenic, since carbonic acid possesses aphrodisiac qualities (just as do extremely cold or warm baths for other patients). Such observations are certainly correct, but their incorporation in medical theory and the attendant emphasis laid unduly upon the significance of sexuality as an aetiological factor appear highly questionable, not to say dissembling. *Pruritus* is no more 'actually' or 'in reality' a state of sexual excitement than the nose or chin are 'actually' male genitals! Just as the chin and the nose are phallic analogies, itching shares a common pruriginous essence with the torment of questions and yearnings related to instinctuality. The Latin word *prurigo*, being used in areas aside from sexuality, implies itching just as much as it does lust or concupiscence. *Prurigo* can also mean the itching of a scab or dandruff, and the related verb *prurire* implies to be desirous of a confrontation, preserved in English as "to be *itching* for a fight."

Itching carries a sense of acute necessity, of something that is 'burning' or 'inflamed' and, therewith, the realm of fire and of the rubbing or friction which starts fires. We hear much the same thing in fire as we do in *pruritus*: crackling, popping, sparking, fizzing, etc. According to legend, when fire is cursed or insulted (in contemporary psychological jargon that would correspond to 'repressing'), it revenges itself through scabs or mange, an 'evil' countenance, or blisters and scales on the tongue or lips. The offender was visited by St. Anthony's fire, by gangrene (an 'eating' or 'burning' sore), or by rose fever, all conditions with a noticeable affinity to fire.

In myths, legends, and fairytales, fire appears as a life form with a wide variety of human forms: a fiery figure, a skeleton with flames shooting out of its ribcage as if it were a burning wicker basket. Sometimes it is gigantic in its proportions, with matchstick legs, or dwarfishly small, often headless with a hollow back and fiery eyes. At other times fire appears as a formless smoldering, a burning bundle of straw, an elusive will-o'-the-wisp darting here and there, or as a wheel of fire, whirring through the air. Our images of fire are countless and carry a certain cross-cultural similarity not only in myths and legends of the past but also in contemporary vernacular, in poetry, and in dreams. Passion, tempers, and lovers, for example, are frequently designated 'fiery.'

Fiery beings in human form are often conceived of as the walking dead atoning for their wickedness in hell's fire, murderers and adulterers forced to live under the ban until the day of deliverance. They seem to represent our asocial or antisocial burnings repressed by collective taboos and condemned to live on in bewitched, perverted form.

The analogous relationship of crackling fire and itching carries over to combustion induced through friction, an activity related to all digging, delving, and scratching. Jung, in his work *Symbols of Transformation*, explores the significance of firemaking, arriving at the hypothesis that the fire-bringing Prometheus is "brother" to the Indian Pramantha, the masculine firestick. Above all, though, it is Agni, god of fire, who springs out of Indian flames, an image which resonates with European hermetical speculations.

In its redeemed form, fire glows in the world's religions as the least delineated, most basic image of the Godhead: as divine love, as Holy Ghost, as mystic radiance, as divine power, or as the light of life itself. We are enlightened when we 'see the light,' and we speak then with 'tongues of fire.' Perhaps, too, in a paroxysm of righteous indignation, we accomplish a stroke of genius, or we are filled with a glowing sense of awe, or we are consumed by the flames of passion. In these states the skin plays a central role: we beam and 'glow.' In the following case study, we will see how such flaming emotions can be concealed in an ordinary, pruriginous dermatosis and how miraculous it seems when what was nothing but a rough and itching malaise recedes to reveal the fiery spirit at its core.

*

The patient in question was not only mentally ill but also suffered from a singular skin condition which varied directly according to her frame of mind. Here and there, but particularly on the extremities, slightly raised splotches, blue-red in color and about the size of a fifty-cent piece, would appear. From time to time they itched severely, finally forming small abscesses in the middle. The exanthema reacted to no medical treatment except for that employed for schizophrenia and cleared up with the appearance of each psychotic episode.

She was the daughter of a clergyman and led something of a scullery-maid existence: she usually ended up with the cleaning and housework as well as responsibility for the garden. No one seemed to remember how this distribution of labor had been arrived at since it only became apparent when her siblings married and left home. There she was with no friends, no career, with no real connection to the outer world, puttering about the house. From that time on, her life became more and more difficult. She became bitter about her fate, developing deep and abiding resentment toward her parents who had raised her in such isolated and miserable conditions. Out of her isolation she began to concoct lofty plans and to transform into something unique but unappreciated.

Since she was so different from her siblings, she believed that she was of noble descent and had been foisted off on her parents. She began collecting postcards of old castles and fortresses and other pictures showing feudal structures. She followed the activities of the remaining marriageable European princes and developed an interest in architecture and the fine arts. Actually, she believed, she was a Gilberte de Courgenay or a Queen Victoria and, following her parents' death, she sponsored needy art and architecture students. When her protégés cheated and exploited her thoroughly, she made shrill cries of protest, but this only served to strengthen her illusions.

When she was filling her inner and outer isolation with feelings of quasi-aristocratic responsibility and enthusiasm, her skin disorder was hardly noticeable. It became acute the moment her delusional reality collapsed, only to vanish into thin air with the outbreak of her almost delirium-like schizophrenic episodes. Then she would hear voices which conversed with her in Oxford English, and she would carry on wondrous dialogues with them. The voices had a magical quality and most certainly came from men, mostly doctors, dentists, and politicians for whom she had felt reverence and affection and who now became delusional lovers. These profane beings became demigods with whom she was in touch "through the air." She imagined that they caressed her, and she went into erotic and sexual ecstasies. Then a sense of nobility and exaltation came to her unbidden: feverishly she wrote about her encounters, about the fountains of wisdom and insight gushing forth from her amorous rendezvous, and she filled page upon page with large script comprising a poetry hardly legible to an outsider.

These ecstasies never reached the point where they interfered with the patient's unpretentious tasks. Aware that her experiences all originated in her, she always maintained a certain degree of control over herself and, therefore, remained free from difficulties with the outer world. The form of her existence remained as unassuming and isolated as it had always been.

*

The subject of itching dermatoses leads us to everything which creeps and crawls, to that which 'bugs' us or makes us 'antsy' or pesters us like a swarm of gnats. Just as *pruritus* combines a condition of dry and crackling discomfort with the inflammation of enthusiasm and erotic stimulation, the logic of folklore links the creeping with the divine. The mythology surrounding vermin of every kind has always been rather ambiguous: it has never been completely negative. The literature which has come down to us on the subject is in no way usurped by accounts of "cerebral animalcules" which account for practically the sum total of psychiatric symptomatology, from passing 'ticks' to the visual hallucinations of psychotic delirium. They are not just simply related to apocalyptic plagues or to animals which announce impending death like the ticking woodworm. The tradition includes much more than merely fear of the repulsive or that which excites itching or that which brings disease. Nor does it end with attempts to bring vermin to trial, as was the case in Lucerne where, in the midst of the plague in 1594, the city council issued a decree to that effect.

On the contrary, the negative qualities of vermin frequently reverse into something reverential, as we have seen how itching gives way to passion and enthusiastic excitement. Such sentiments and notions are especially found with creatures living in the most degrading environments: the dung beetle and its relatives are a prime example. These insects maintain their existence and derive nourishment from the manure of domestic animals and are designated in almost every language according to their habitat. By the hundreds they scramble around on dung heaps, especially when the surface has been dried out by the heat of the sun and, with the help of their wings, they assay occasional, short, humming flights. As wretched as the conditions of this world sometimes appear and as miserable as the existence of the dung beetle seems, so has its shimmering luster excited fantasies of something exquisite or even holy.

The dung beetle is as much related to *pruritus* as the crackling fire is: at least in legends it is linked to storm deities like the Germanic god Thor, and in some regions it is believed that stepping on a dung beetle invites a lightning fire. It magically produces sparkling treasures and, in Kernten, putting a dung beetle in a safe-deposit box is supposed to guarantee a never-ending source of money. When innocent children look into brand-new, shiny, copper pots swarming with dung beetles, they can see the reflection of shiny coins. In places where money has been seen burning, dung beetles are later found. It is not surprising that the *geotrupes stercorarius* (*stercus* 'manure,' 'excrement') was considered a *spiritus familiaris*, like the toad in the cellar which in folklore was left a saucer of milk.

The dung beetle has achieved its ultimate exaltation, though, in a zoological relative, namely, the scarab beetle or *ateuchus sacer*. The scarab, too, dwells in dung and was considered so holy by the Egyptians that it was embalmed upon its death. It was assumed that the scarab, termed the "self-generated one," emerged from primordial mud or primal dung as the first being on earth, a manifestation of the god of gods, Atum, whose name is equivalent to "The Nothing." After Atum became identified with the highest sun god, the scarab was correspondingly regarded as a miniaturized, fiery Ra. It is a paradox without equal, a chimera of meanings like those of disease syndromes viewed not from the perspective of natural science but through the lenses of the archetypes.

*

A continual process of somatization takes place just below the surface of our consciousness, taking on forms which at first are not readily recognizable for what they are. This holds true for itching, *pruritus*, where the degree of acuteness seems to be directly correlated with the extent to which a kind of isolation capacity interrupts an openness to one's environment. It is just this capacity for isolation which modern civilization depends on: the more industrialized a society is, the more certainly the isolation capacity is functioning.

Today this capacity has assumed more subtle forms which we designate as hygiene and cosmetics, both of which, without our really being aware of it, have taken on something of the nature of religious cults. We practice them as matter-of-factly as we earlier did the rituals of the church, and even excesses go unnoticed because of their collective quality. At best we become aware of the phenomena after the fact, as history, or when some reformer is struck by the horror of it all.

As was the case with earlier rituals, those surrounding our dealings with the skin are becoming more and more differentiated. Daily libations of soap and water have long given way to more complex ceremonies: salves are daubed on from a cornucopic palette of chemical substances, facial masks are plastered on indiscriminately, morning and evening the skin is 'nourished' and kept 'moist.' Various procedures supposedly open and close the pores and much, much more.

The assertion has been made that these chemical substances are responsible for an overwhelming increase in the incidence of skin disorders. If dermatoses have, in point of fact, assumed epidemic proportions, the causes are not nearly as certain as is sometimes maintained. It would seem, rather, that chemical substances merely serve as a vehicle, as the means to an end, whereby repressed, socially unreconciled emotionality attempts to break out of an imposed isolation. It would seem that the increase in dermatoses lives more from a collective compulsion toward isolation and loneliness and less from contact with heretofore unknown, artificial substances.

Cardiac Dysrhythmia

LIKE other muscular organs—the intestines or the ureter, for example—the heart possesses a relative autonomy. The impulse for heartbeats originates in the sinus node, a kind of natural pacemaker which, in human beings, is located at the point where the superior vena cava opens into the right atrium. The impulse then spreads through the atrial walls where the musculature, like that of the heart as a whole, is comprised of two different kinds of muscle fibers or, rather, of muscle cells. Those which are predominantly striated and fibrillose contract and generate tension and, in their entirety, are designated the working myocardium. Passing through and contracting the atria, the impulse reaches a second node, the atrioventricular node, located on the wall between the atria where the right atrium and right ventricle meet. It then proceeds into the His' Bundle, a conductive tissue layer running along the septum between the ventricles to the apex of the heart where it fans out. In this manner the impulse proceeds from the sinus node through the entire heart so that the musculature contracts at the appropriate moment.

It is noteworthy that the rhythm of the heartbeat becomes slower and slower in the latter stages of the above process when the orderly progression is interfered with either artificially or as the result of disease. Independent of any outside influence, the sinus node operates at a rate of sixty to eighty beats per minute as opposed to the atrioventricular node's rate of fifty to sixty beats per minute. Different autorhythms also exist in the His'

Bundle: we speak of a "bundle rhythm" of between twenty-five and forty-five beats per minute. Under normal circumstances the autonomy of the heart is but a relative one, heart functions being influenced significantly by the autonomous nervous system. The autonomous nervous system affects not only the pulse rate but also the sensitivity to stimulus and strength of the heart. The nerves of the sympathetic nervous system have their origin in the upper part of the thoracic area of the spinal cord, while the vagus nerve is the primary agent of the parasympathetic nervous system. The sympathetic system stimulates heart functions; the parasympathetic system inhibits them. Even the autonomous nervous system is only relatively autonomous and its point of origin in the brain stem simply a network with connections in all directions.

*

Generally speaking, the heartbeat is a temperate occurrence and follows a set pattern. However, there are characteristic exceptions, phenomena called "fibrillations" and "fluttering," "racing" or "stumbling," all combined under the heading of "cardiac dysrhythmia." Although the pulse rate of a trained athlete gives one the impression of stoic imperturbability, not exceeding a sinus rhythm of sixty to seventy beats per minute even under physical exertion, the above-mentioned disturbances give the impression of total chaos. Dysrhythmia occur in those who are 'healthy' as well as those with a history of heart conditions. It is a disease, a syndrome which, following the perspective of archetypal medicine, assumes varying degrees or levels of somatization and correspondingly varying degrees of seriousness. They might be passing electrophysiological caprices leaving no noticeable traces in the anatomy of the cardiac wall. On the other hand, they may cause changes in the myocardia—visible under the microscope or even to the naked eye—which reveal themselves as scars and tissue degeneration on the autopsy table.

Another element which corresponds to the pathogenetic conceptions of archetypal medicine is that cardiac dysrhythmia are most unselective as to causal agents. Noxae of any sort seem to suffice nicely: a disagreement at work or an argument at home, a declaration of love or of ill-will. Stormy weather or excessive amounts of nicotine or caffeine set the stage for rhythmic disorders as much as does a reduction in the blood supply to the myocardium from sclerosis of the coronary arteries or viral and bacterial myocarditis, an inflammation of the heart muscles.

Where heart fibrillations and flutters occur, the heartbeat may get as high as 250 to 300 beats per minute, a circumstance which can cause death when the ventricles are affected but which may go unnoticed when the dysrhythmia are limited to the atria. Patients may complain of unusual discomforts, or being a bit dizzy or lightheaded, or of a constricted feeling around the heart. Occasionally they may lose consciousness: the extent and severity of the complaints depend on how well the various organs are supplied with blood. In cases of paroxysmal tachycardia, the heartbeat is not as high, usually around 140. The condition is nevertheless experienced as a 'racing' of the heart, although the pulse is flat and barely discernible. Due to the resulting constrictions which sometimes occur, the patient may be short of breath, feel lightheaded, or appear pale, while organs such as the liver and the lungs may be congested because of insufficient circulation.

In addition to conditions of increased heartbeat, all of which are rhythmic, there are also the so-called "arrhythmia," irregularities, in short, of the sequence of heart contractions. Clinically, the most significant of these is heart "stumbling" or extrasystole, where the beats occur out of sequence with an extended pause from one to the next. To the patient it seems as if the heart had stopped, causing fear or giving rise to the lascivious sense that a version of Russian roulette is being played. When the pause between beats is extended and the extrasystoles increase, the patient has the impression that his

heart is being strangled or that he is close to losing consciousness.

*

The etymology of a phenomenon is often suited to move from
a medically objective perspective to an immediate and experiential one. The verbs used to characterize cardiac rhythmic disturbances imply increased activity on the one hand and the
nearness of death on the other. The German equivalent of
"fibrillation," *flimmer* 'a flickering,' is related to the English
word "flame," the Latin *flamma* and *flagrare*, 'blazing' or 'glowing,' with the Greek *phlogmos* 'flame,' *phlegma* 'blaze,' or with
the Latvian *blazma* 'glimmer' or 'gleam.' The term "flutter" is
connected to "flare" but also to the German *Fledermaus* 'bat,' a
"fluttering" mouse. We hear not only the helpless fluttering of a
bird or a moth but also the relationship between "mouse" and
"muscle" and, thereby, to the myocardium, a relationship
which is clearly expressed in the Latin *mus*, meaning 'mouse'
and 'muscle.' It would seem that there is not only a medical comprehension but a medical *appre*hension, an intuition arising
from the consanguinity of all things.

The etymology of "racing," from a "racing of the heart," leads
to borderline conditions. The Anglo-Saxon *raes* 'race' also
means 'to attack' and 'to storm,' and *rasettan* is a 'rage.' *Rasettan*
contains the Indo-Germanic root *ras*, meaning 'a raging stream'
or 'rapids.' It is not surprising that during the Rhenish carnival
season the Monday before Ash Wednesday is called *Rosenmon-
tag* (literally "Rose Monday," but where *Rosen* refers not to a
variety of flowers but to the dialect pronunciation of the verb
rasen 'to race'). Luther used the word "race" in place of "rave" to
mean 'being beside oneself.'

Where "stuttering" and heart stutters are concerned, there is a
connection to "stammer" and, through the Norwegian *stumla*,
to "stumble," the German *stolpern* 'stumble,' and to the Swedish
stjälpa 'fall' or 'collapse.' It would seem that when our hearts
"stutter" we stumble and fall.

*

In the context of archetypal medicine, cardiac dysrhythmia can be understood as varying forms of being 'beside oneself.' Generally occurring as paroxysms, they are emotional seizures which find their expression primarily in the body because other outlets are denied them. The body gives expression to what otherwise would be passion, a fluttery anxiety, a racing rage, a sense of transcendence, or simply the occasional chaos of emotionality that is part of human experience. It is as if we fall apart or come to a fall when emotions 'descend' into body and make themselves felt as disease syndromes of indeterminate origin. It is as if cardiac dysrhythmia catch us in an alien web with surrealistic overtones.

Also corresponding to the pathogenetic concepts of archetypal medicine is the fact that, the more we are unknowingly dominated by the fantasy of harmony, the greater the incidence of dysrhythmia. Cardiac disturbances intrude on our lives particularly when we matter-of-factly believe in a harmonic togetherness, when we assume that a mother's warm heart or a father's kindly heart beats out the time of our existence. Just where we unquestioningly attempt to fulfill our obligations to notions of harmony, something foreign, something disharmonious, breaks in upon us, jeopardizing our entire Weltanschauung.

*

A fear or phobia of heart conditions or heart attacks is a superficial somatization of being 'beside oneself,' experienced as a sudden racing of the heart accompanied by an increase in blood pressure and rapid, shallow breathing. The afflicted patient fears for his very life, fears that his heart will literally stop beating. He never loses consciousness, though, even when the situation appears apocalyptic and lasts for over an hour at a time. He feels like his heart is beating all over his body. Shaken as he is, he can hardly escape the fear (even during the intervals) that the next seizure is imminent and will cost him his life. Consequently, he tries to remain as near as he can to doctors, from whom he can expect lifesaving attention.

In industrialized nations, heart phobias are as common in their occurrence as they are limited in the degree of somatization and are treated accordingly by psychosomatic medicine. The phobias occur predominantly among those who are only children and whose relationships to their parents or teachers have been ambivalent. The group includes orphans and half-orphans as well as the youngest children in a family who, even in later life, exist in a kind of *participation mystique* and who, in other words, never grow out of the ambivalence of a love-hate relationship. It would seem that their 'hearts' wished to beat in rhythm with those of others out of a preconscious claim or demand for attention. At the same time, there seems to be some 'thing' which would light up the darkness of this sort of infantile unconsciousness with a stroke of lightning, as if Nature would destroy this measure of order with her ordering immeasurability.

*

Here is a case in point. She was an affectionate, sincere, devoted, and responsible only-child with a pretty, cherubic face. She smiled as if the heart of the whole world were delight and enjoyment. At the same time she had a high, almost resolute voice, and her heartiness became rather loud on occasions. At the age of twenty she was still very much a girl.

Her heart attacks began after her German shepherd died of cancer. She had spent most of her youth and adolescence with him and was as devoted to the dog as she would have been to a brother or sister. From time to time she was overcome by a sudden fear: her heart raced and stumbled and seemed to her as if it were full of holes. Her entire body would tremble and perspire. The attack passed after a half hour, leaving her exhausted and disgusted with herself. Whenever her heartbeat varied from the accustomed rhythm, it seemed that her world was coming to an end. The intervals between the attacks were, themselves, not free of symptoms: she snacked compulsively, particularly on sweets, becoming rounder and rounder despite futile attempts to fast for days at a time.

She grew up on the shores of one of the Swiss lakes in an older house with a garden that ran down to the water's edge. Everything was well-ordered and in a state of relative well-being, financially as well as domestically. Her father traded cattle and was a jovial man who made others laugh. Her mother preached an ideology of self-discipline and was not the kind of person who readily fell apart. As she grew up, the patient became accustomed to the notion that everything had to have its proper place and that she could be of one heart and mind with everything around her. There were various ways in which 'Nature' attempted to censure these pre- or unconscious assumptions: a sense of impending storm and a sudden drop in temperature when she was taken by a chill or when she learned of a death in the neighborhood or read the expression "taken from us" in the obituaries. What bothered her most of all were those emotional responses from her boyfriend which seemed or might have indicated a turning away from her on his part. Consequently, she watched over him jealously, clung to him, and sorely tested his patience. It is somewhat surprising that her jealousy did not achieve the opposite of what she had intended and that he did end up marrying her. Due as much to his patience and understanding as to her psychotherapy, the patient's attacks disappeared after three years, and she had no further complaints. Her therapy concentrated on a revaluation of the state of being 'beside oneself,' on discovering a greater trust in her manifold 'hysterias,' and on insights into the relative nature of her idealized *harmonia mundi*.

*

In the course of her psychotherapy, the patient volunteered for an experiment in sleep and dream research, but her participation was to no avail because of her insomnia or, rather,

her anxiety. The surroundings seemed too cold, too scientific to her and, after only one night, the experiment had to be called off. Nonetheless, during one short interval of sleep, she had a pathognomonic dream which lent itself admirably to an amplification and understanding of her "heart racing." In the dream she was half human, half monster, lying in the bed in the research laboratory. Here and there, especially on her arms and legs, she was covered with scales. In place of her normal feet she had prehensile ones with which she could hold fast to the foot of the bed. Seeing them, she awoke appalled, her heart beating wildly at 130 beats per minute.

Understanding this dream presupposes knowledge of a vast, somewhat ill-defined species of 'birds.' We might begin with the Harpies and related birds of prey which, according to Homer, were the "goddesses of sweeping storms and of death," while Hesiod considered them to be hybrids, a cross between human maidens and birds of prey. They, too, had armored skin and claws which closed like machines around everything that came within their reach. One of the most vivid accounts of these beings is found in the *Aeneid*. Following their defeat at the hands of the Greeks, the fleeing Trojans found themselves on an island inhabited by a swarm of Harpies who considered it theirs. Constantly pale and gray from hunger, these creatures fell with the suddenness of a summer storm upon any and all nourishment which anyone else tried to eat. Their assault was accompanied by murderous screams, by the fouling of everything with filth, and by the unbearable stench which they left behind. Their visitation was truly an attack, a seizure, a fluttering, a racing, and a horror.

There are a number of parallels between the Harpies and this patient, not only in their maidenly qualities but also in their relationship to food which we may here see as signifying security and protection, something to hold on to which guaranteed a quasi-mystical sense of participation with everything. The Harpies reached as inevitably for food as did the patient for her snacks: they could no more ignore food than she could, without flying into a rage or becoming terribly anxious. While the Harpies left stench and excrement behind, the patient was left with a disgust of herself.

In many ways the Harpies are related to the Sirens, whose charms find such prominence in poetry: the irresistible quality of their songs and flutes as well as their insatiability. They, too, are usually winged, and, in addition to having the heads of maidens, they have claws to slay their victims. When Ulysses sailed past their island, all that remained to be seen of their prey was bones, gnawed and picked clean, on the beach.

Vampires and other types of blood-sucking parasites also belong to the family of such bird-like creatures whose members have inhabited the earth since the beginning of time. They, too, are usually pale from their hunger for blood and, instead of fingernails, they have claws. They, too, are possessed by a bloodthirsty dependence on their victims and can only be kept away by having stakes driven through their hearts and being buried.

Finally, Harpies, Sirens, and Vampires are also related to the Germanic Valkyries, those virgins of the battlefield who bore off the slain but who also spread paralyzing fear among the warriors. Valkyries are a variety of woodland bird, similar to crows, but to whom fantasy has attributed erotic powers. For the Vikings they not only announced the coming of death but served also in Valhalla as "Odin's maidens" or prostitutes. They brought their victims to the peak of honor. They have been called nymphs by historians or *virgines silvestres*, wood-nymphs, who tempt men to their death with their beauty. Always, though, there was an accompanying flutter, a storming, and an intoxication. It seems as if nothing out of the ordinary can take place without the heart deviating from its measured rhythm.

Amplifying the theme of harmony and disruption leads to Orpheus and Pythagoras, both imbued with a faith in the musical euphony of existence and both who, in their own respective fashions, suffered the fate of sudden devastation. According to tradition, one was torn apart by maenads while the other saw his temple burned to the ground.

Orpheus was an extraordinary singer and could fascinate one and all with his lyre. Not only could he move the very rocks and boulders, but also he could tame wild animals who normally would have devoured each other. Because of his musical ability the Argonauts took him along on their voyage: he knew how to calm the storms with his playing and how to drown out the deathly song of the Sirens. His ability is not so surprising considering his parentage, for noble Apollo was his father and the muse Calliope, "she of the beautiful voice," his mother. Usually, though, Calliope is portrayed as a lyricist, with tablet and stylus in hand.

As well as Orpheus knew how to produce harmony wherever he went, a kind of 'loving togetherness,' so to speak, and a sense of the coherence of life, he just as unavoidably was met with the loss of his wife Euridice. Thanks to his music, he almost succeeded in retrieving her from the underworld and would have had he not broken his agreement not to turn around to see if she were still following him. He became suddenly afraid that he had been cheated. The shock and bitter disappointment of the event had serious consequences for him: from that time on he avoided all women, withdrawing into the forests of Greece where he became a legend. There he led a relatively homophilious, misogynous life, appearing in early Christian descriptions as Christ and the Good Shepherd. It is as if, following his fateful experience, he sought more than ever to give voice to the old faith and as if the danger of a catastrophic end became even more pronounced. Nature goes to considerable effort to insure that we do not confuse the universe with an idyll!

Although Orpheus was not afflicted with jealous Harpies and did not vanish as the victim of vampires, he was torn to pieces by the maenads, women who, at dionysian festivals, go into ecstasies, become 'beside themselves,' and rage through the Thracian forests murdering and raping. The name "maenad" is connected to "mania," to madness, in other words, and therefore the maenads are similar in nature to the Harpies. Orpheus was not killed merely by the "natural/physical," as oversimplifying mythologists would have it, but primarily by Nature's unpredictable eruptions and spontaneities.

Because he is mythological, Orpheus is also immortal: his fate is a universal, human one, and his conflict, between harmony and madness, belongs to each of us in one form or another. We can also understand why the story of Orpheus did not remain only a legend but became the central theme of a cult, the Orphic sect, which is also related to the cult of Dionysos who, himself, was dismembered by the maenads. The Orphics were almost pantheistic, inclining to the belief that everything came into being out of the heart of Zeus and owed its existence to him. As an expression of their need to affirm the oneness of all things, they did away with polytheism and installed Zeus as the supreme God of the universe. The Orphic mysteries were bloody and rested upon the perception that all forms of being 'beside oneself,' of chaos, belong to the rhythm and harmony of the heart.

Pythagoras was a later Orphic who, like Orpheus himself, dealt with the measured and the temperate and, consequently, with the measured beat of the heart as well. The lyre, which as we know is usually heart-shaped, possessed a definite significance for him, too. He found that, by keeping the tension constant and varying the length of the strings, he could create a musical scale, a fact which he proceeded to translate into the ordering of the entire universe according to fixed proportions. Subsequently, he developed the concept of a world harmony. He heard the music of the spheres (imperceptible to others) in which Concordia, accord, was perceptible; he regarded the earth as a ball, floating in the cosmos and encased by the orbits of sun and planets.

Living in Sicily, among other places, during the second half of the sixth century B. C., Pythagoras founded a kind of order in Croton which spread his teachings concerning world harmony.

That which was possessed of measure was raised to the position of ultimate norm. In general, the members followed strict dietary requirements and ate simply of wholesome food, depending upon what was to be had, what one had a right to, and what conformed with principles of moral-religious instructions and self-control. The order obtruded to such an extent on the rest of the island and gained so much political influence that it evoked its own annihilation: the Temple of the master was put to the torch and burned to the ground. It seemed as if so much harmony could not exist without compelling the fire of passion to consume it.

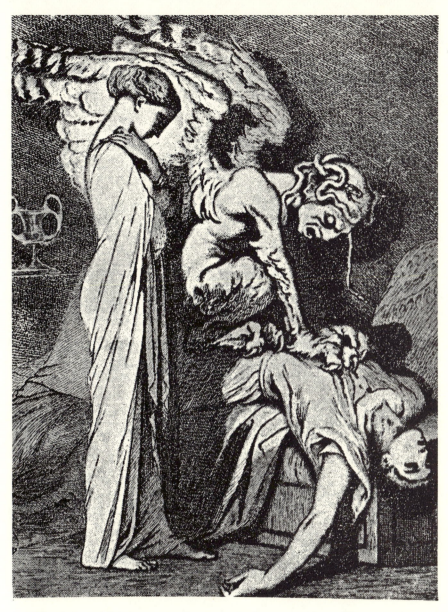

The beautiful Meroe as the vampire's accomplice. Illustration from "Smarra or the Demon of the Night" by Charles Nodier. Wherever the state of being 'beside oneself' occurs as a rhythmic disturbance of the heart, archetypal medicine makes associations to that mythical genus of winged creatures which is traditionally characterized by its fascination as well as by its qualities of terror-spreading hysteria.

Anorexia Nervosa

THERE exists a trait peculiar to living things which apparently appears exclusively in human beings and then in a unique manner sometimes bordering on the grotesque. It is a trait which we will call the ascetic instinct. This instinct sets itself against a number of natural impulses, against hunger, for example, or against gregarious tendencies or the desire for possession, against sexual cupidity and egoistic self-indulgence, against laziness and the need for verbal communication. In general this instinct sets itself against the world of the material wherever the material is manifested as formlessness or shapelessness. Wherever this ascetic instinct appears, it has a generalized effect and, under normal circumstances, serves to preserve the contours, the shape and form, of human nature.

The term "ascetic" originally meant 'exercise,' *exercitium*, the preparation, by moderation in lifestyle and physical training, of Greek athletes for competition. It was adapted by several schools of philosophy—the Pythagoreans, the Cynics, and the Stoics—for whom it became a characteristic way of life. The natural ascetic instinct came to play an increasingly important part in human behavior and began increasingly to be attributed an ethical significance as a means of overcoming bad habits and vices. Man's sense of himself became more and more discordant. More than ever before he seemed to be possessed by a kind of dualism: his physical nature, against which asceticism was directed, was frequently regarded as the object of disgust, as a "prison of the soul." Freeing oneself from this primal slime or mud could only be regarded as the highest virtue.

Throughout the history of Christian Europe, the almost mythical image of release from the body made its appearance under varying conditions. As Ludwig Tieck expressed it in romantic fashion: "Wie ein freigemachter Vogel soll die Seele in den reinen, blauen Himmel der Wahrheit und Unschuld hineinflattern, um in klarem Licht zu schwimmen." ("Like a bird set free, let the soul wing its way into the pure, blue heaven of truth and innocence, to swim in the clarity of light.") We can understand this vision as a thoroughly natural one, especially when the individual in question is groaning under the weight of his own obesity and despairs in the face of his unbridled appetite, when his respect in the community is destroyed due to his lechery and he is driven to thoughts of suicide because of a compulsion to masturbate, or when his conscience eats away at him because he neglects his work out of an irresistible laziness. Under such circumstances, a sojourn in the "blue heaven of truth and innocence" might well seem the noblest and most desirable goal, a place where existence becomes the purity of the spirit.

The history of ascetic behavior and thinking began at the end of an era which had a completely different perspective. For a period which must have lasted for well over a hundred thousand years, the focus of religious belief seems to have been a mother deity unsurpassable in corpulence and ponderance. During this stone age, mankind revered the very things which later asceticism so abhorred. The cultic stone figures of this obese deity can be found from Siberia to the Pyrenees, an area, in other words, which includes present-day Europe. It is astonishing that the objects of this form of worship and the Weltanschauung to which they bear witness did not owe their widespread existence to the migration of tribes and races but seem to have sprung up autochthonously and simultaneously from the earth. The general worship of an Earth Mother figure is, therefore, not basically different from that given other archetypal principals within the history of mankind, such as the image of the wounded, suffering god.

The appearance or, rather, the shape of these primal mother or feminine cult-figures often borders on the grotesque: the trunk is extremely full and corpulent, the posterior formed into overwhelmingly fatty buttocks (steatopygia). The figures seem to point to the position of reverence accorded eating and the material in general, including possessions. The majority of the figures give the impression of pregnancy, emphasizing the value placed on fertility and reproduction, while the heads by contrast are relatively small and indicate the low esteem in which things of the intellect or spirit were held. The arms, held tightly against the body and sometimes not even clearly separated from it, as well as the legs, which give the impression of being one rather than two and end in tiny feet, convey the sense of an oppressive heaviness and immobility, even of paralysis. The breasts seem bursting with fullness, and the genital region is almost always characterized by a marked prominence of the pubic hair, the labia, or the genital opening, indicating the supreme significance of sexuality. All of these biological instincts revered through the stone-age, feminine cult-figures became to varying degrees the object of later taboos. The stagnation and unhistorical character of the megalithic world found an end in the gradual spread of an ascetic self-image.

In anorexia nervosa the instinct for the ascetic takes possession of the individual, frequently in absurdly exaggerated intensity, and its effect is always total. All aspects of biological instinctuality revered in antiquity are indiscriminately subjected to restrictions. We can understand why the clinical picture—the repetitive, relatively typical lifestyle—of the anorectic corresponds, if somewhat exaggeratedly, in many ways to the ethical stance idealized by Neoplatonic philosophy and Christianity. Both Neoplatonism and Christianity set limits to and for the purely biological. Consequently, the term "anorexia" is fallacious since not only ingestion of nutrients is restricted but other biological drives as well. The taboo placed on eating is only one of the various ascetic practices, even if it is the most dangerous. As an entity, anorexia is directed toward the goal when she is finished. Usually those around the anorectic refuse to stand by passively and watch as she dwindles to a shadow of her former self. For this reason the anorectic feels watched and develops various ways to camouflage her actions such as lying, hiding, and making promises. When anorectics do indeed eat, they prefer foods which are low in calories, foods with little nutritional value and which do not give a feeling of heaviness or contribute to weight gain. Anorectics especially avoid fats, since fat for them is associated with everything which is amorphous and formlessly steatopygic—stinking, sweating fleshiness. They much prefer lemons, green apples, and other similar forms of 'non-nourishing' nutrition.

Anorectics often prefer to eat alone, a sign of their propensity for solitude which, although not a source of suffering, points to their hermit tendencies. Consequently, mealtimes are not regarded as a time for togetherness and closeness and are often as sparse as the anorectic's lettuce salad or as sour as a vinegar-and-oil dressing. The table conversation, though, can often be quite stimulating or, on the other hand, narrow-minded and fanatic. Anorectics do not look to dinners, even large, holiday feasts, for a sense of warm humanity, especially not when the Thanksgiving or Christmas tables are laden with meats, gravies, and alcohol, an experience they find repulsive. That which is all-too-human and intimate generally nauseates them. It is this ready feeling of nausea which acts as a guard against life's materialism, something that non-anorectics do not experience. Although anorectics try to remain above their nausea, it is not uncommon for them to rid themselves of what they have eaten by self-induced vomiting. This could be viewed as an attempt at a sort of 'de-materialization.' To avoid putting on weight and an attendant identification with steatopygic, amorphous human-ity, they also use large quantities of purgatives and even diuretics. By being increasingly 'above-it-all,' anorectics add to their own sense of 'weight' or importance and subsequently to the friction and buffeting from those around them, but in no wise do they contribute to the sought-after qualities of the spiritual and ethereal.

Another instinct which falls under the dominance of the ascetic drive is that of movement: anorectics avoid laziness, sometimes sleep as well, and take extended walks, although it is difficult to imagine how their emaciated bodies ever manage to get out the door. Activity is not primarily a means of losing weight but more a manifestation of the compulsion to avoid succumbing to the sluggishness and inertia of the gravitational pull of all that is earthly. If the anorectic employs appetite-reducing medication as well, the compulsion is simply magnified since hardly any of these drugs fail to increase motoric activity. The drugs themselves are generally 'ascetic.'

As far as their abiding denial of rest and materialism is concerned, anorectics seem to have re-instituted Christian and pre-Christian practices which were especially common among hermits and monastics. They, too, seem to have availed themselves of 'ascetic' drugs. In his work, *Concerning the Raising of the Dead, as well as Unusually Extended Sleeping and Fasting*, Agrippa of Nettesheim reports herbs which even in the smallest doses allow extensive fasting. He cites as examples Nicholas of Fluellen and Elijah, although it is recorded that the latter was supplied with bread and other food by ravens during his time in the desert. Christian virtue is also expressed by anorectics inasmuch as they often apply their seemingly excessive energies for altruistic purposes: they like to help others even to the extent of cooking for them!

'De-materialization,' that process by which anorectics escape all aspects of Mother Earth, is not only visible in the guise of physical emaciation but in more subtle forms as well: the basic metabolic rate declines, body temperature falls, heartbeat and breathing are slowed, and blood pressure decreases. This extensive reduction of basic life processes is not accompanied by any suffering but, quite to the contrary, seems connected to a kind of triumphant cheerfulness! It seems to serve as a curious testimonial to a gigantic defiance dwelling in living beings, a challenge to and a denial of gods and Nature, which only in human beings appears to assume such saint-like qualities. The ascetic instinct is terroristic and its satisfaction found in the demise of the material and the non-spiritual. Approximately twenty percent of anorectic patients die, after having experienced the "pure and blue" of heaven and tasted, through their denial of life, of its freedom from suffering.

*

And yet the anorectic's satisfaction is never 'pure.' It is interrupted by disgruntlement, by the feeling of being surrounded by a vacuum, by disappointments and nagging questions, by discontent and doubts, and most of all by a wide range of varying demands. In fact, it seems to be these very things which interrupt that are responsible for calling forth and maintaining the anorectic or ascetic. Without gluttony, without greed in general, there would be no asceticism.

It is as if the denial of the material, physical greed is the very thing which forces anorexia to take on physical form. To satisfy their demands, anorectics will not even stop short of extortion: they torment those around them and particularly those to whom they have emotional ties—their parents, for example, their spouses, their doctors. They seem to be driven by wishes and desires which they are unable to put into words. They blame others and extenuating circumstances for their plight so that, initially, they are taken at their word. In time, however, their credibility decreases as the addictive nature of their expectations becomes apparent.

The ascetic ideal, therefore, is always intertwined with its opposite, a colossal demand, a *hunger* for something inexpressible. It is this hunger, contrasting so strikingly with the usual feigned selflessness, which finds its expression in rebellious egotism, in always trying to get the upper hand, in narcissistic egocentricity, as well as in the eating habits discussed above. Anorectics are a continual source of amazement in the way they unexpectedly devour food and in their inventiveness in playing games of hide-and-seek with those who simply want to help them toward a more rational nutrition. Seen over a period of time, even their activity becomes questionable, more a running in place than actually accomplishing anything, less of an actual change in the anorectics and their life and more of a "much ado" about an unchanging "nothing." There exists little, if any, developmental or fundamental change: their ideas remain stiff and unmoving, monotonously uniform or unbendingly fanatic. Changes which do occur are only superficial, and the earthy heaviness they so compulsively flee overtakes them in the form of 'eternal' monotony. Although they take great pains with the aid of purgatives and laxatives to rid themselves of all the food that they take in, they are otherwise reserved, holding covetously to everything they have.

*

The paradoxes observed in other areas of anorectic asceticism also occur in conjunction with sexual temperance and innocence: anorectics avoid the theme of sexuality as much as they do that of food and eating. At best they talk about the difficulties they have with their spouses. Sexuality can be forgotten to such an extent that it becomes literally nonexistent, regressing, so to speak, to the time prior to menarche and where all further development is arrested. Menstruation ceases or never begins, so that sexuality remains under the aegis of virginity or girlishness. On the other hand, this innocence and modesty are often distorted into obscenity by licentious thoughts and practices. Anorectics act as if the words "whore" and "nun" were synonymous for them, an attitude which corresponds to earlier concepts of convent-dwellers.

In cities of the Franconian Empire, for example, it was female pilgrims, of all people, who paid homage to a *venus vulgivaga*, a kind of ubiquitously wandering love goddess. At the time of the

the associations to it and their import are, like those of the snake, operative in uncanny, even grotesque ways. Why should we be afraid of toads, why should we sense revulsion for them, and why, especially, are anorectics revulsed by toads, creatures which tend to be awkward, slimy, formless, and blubbery? To answer these questions, we have to realize to what extent the ascetic instincts have come to dominate our consciousness and how, through revulsion, anxiety, and shock, they hold our more primitive and primal instincts in check. Toads were considered to be inordinately gluttonous, partially because of their wide mouths and the 'sticky' tongues with which they greedily pulled in insects and other small amphibians. Witches and creatures associated with them took on the form of toads, according to folklore, and, as such, took part in black sabbaths or sucked milk out of cows' udders as they stood in their stalls.

When hungry, the toad became wild and unruly; as womb or uterus, that which births and mothers, it was a living, self-sufficient being. As womb it demanded sexual satisfaction. Otherwise, it turned into a penis-hungry monster moving restlessly about in the body, causing all sorts of physical complaints particularly in the stomach. Intestinal noises were heard to be its 'cooing,' and its movements could clearly be followed beneath the abdominal wall. This perverted behavior served as the explanation for hysteriform (Greek *hysteros* 'womb') and other kinds of physical disorders. In a way, such superstitions are confirmed by the behavior of the anorectic, whose thoughts and fantasies seem to be guided by them. Anorectics are known for their hypochondriacal attention to everything occurring in the region of the stomach and abdomen. They feel like they have overeaten even though objectively there is no reason for it. Every sensation from the abdominal region is registered immediately as nausea-producing. This gives the impression that anorectics are unable to come to terms with their abdominal organs where so much that is 'vegetative' takes place and which of all organs are more closely related to a world where frogs and toads are at home. For them, the world is still populated by "bufonids" (Latin *bufo* 'toad'), amorphous monsters, gluttonous and lecherous, which undermine and call a world of ethereal spirituality into question.

In Switzerland toads are regarded as domestic spirits. This seems to testify to a certain psychological wisdom, a kind of profound 'arrangement' with everything that is despised. The toads lived in the cellars and were fed daily with a few drops of milk or milk-foam from a silver spoon. They were said to live up to twenty years in the same house and, according to legend, saw to it that the inhabitants never wanted for well-being or money.

Everywhere in legends and myths, we are reminded how necessary it is to have an attitude of kindness and benevolence toward toads, for behind their ugliness and coarseness, behind their common, uncoordinated hopping and silly stare, they conceal a beneficial *daimon* of vegetation. Sometimes they demand one or even three kisses to be released from their reviled existence which, understood symbolically, would be a healing conversion for the anorectic. Usually, however, anorectics persevere throughout their lives in an unchanging, ascetic attitude toward everything which appears so directly appealing in the symbolism of the toad.

Rheumatism
Of Joints and Stiffening

NATURE plays a profound game with flexibility and rigidity. It is as if she audaciously mixed these principles and released different shapes to provide even more multifaceted proofs of her fantasy. It is as if hers were the pleasure of a playwright, watching her own works dance, gesticulate, rush, stiffen, and become crippled. It is as if she had broken the bones of her creations, converting the fractures to joints as these breaks threaten to ossify. It is as if there, where flexibility could have become frenzy, she inserted stability and stubbornness.

The concept is by no means new. The mystic image of being engulfed by flexibility and rigidity seems to have already engaged the minds of the pre-Christian era. This vision takes on shape primarily in Hinduism's pantheon. One is particularly reminded of those gods who, like Shiva, perform a multi-limbed dance in a wheel of flickering fire upon a prostrate corpse. It is just those gods who hold the power over destruction and healing, over the ability to separate and to consolidate.

Etymologically we find the Indo-Germanic root *kleng* 'to bend or to flex' in all articulation. In this root it is not difficult to hear something onomatopoeic which recurs as the "links" of a chain and in the Latin *cingere* 'to be girded with a chain.' It is found in the Middle High German *Gelenke* originally signifying the flexible part between the ribs and the pelvis. Therefore, it appears that the root was used initially to designate the hip-joint, the lumbar region, or the "flank": *lanke* in Middle High German, just as *lanca* in Old High German, meant 'the hip.' *Kleng* is also found in the German *lenken* 'to direct, to turn,' whereby flexibility takes on the quality of being steered, controlled, implying a certain limitation of freedom.

On the other hand, we find the root *stip* in "stiff," as in stiffening of the joints. It probably meant 'rigid' originally but also 'stake' and 'stick.' In Middle High German it becomes *stif*, again 'stiff,' but also 'stately' and 'stare' in which the fixed quality of the seeing is underlined. In Old Norse, *stifr* meant 'unbending,' reappearing in German as *Stift* 'an independent institution.' *Stip* is also found in the Latin *stipes*, which means much the same thing as 'stem,' in the sense of 'originating from' as from a race or a people, botanically as a trunk or plant 'stem,' i.e., something with a high degree of continuity. In other words, everything which is derived from *stip* is not only immovable but also steadfast.

Starting with "stare," a rigid gaze, and the rigidity of an ankylosed joint, what we are doing becomes more obvious. In "stare" we find the root *ster* 'stiffness.' In Gothic it changes to *staurran* and in German to *stoerrisch*, both meaning 'stubborn,' 'recalcitrant.' That the root is also found in the German *sterben* 'to die' is attributable to the fact that the deceased succumbs to or lapses into the rigidity of rigor mortis, staring stubbornly into space. Finally, the root is also found in the German *Storren* 'treetrunk,' in which the aspect of inflexibility and steadfastness is again pronounced.

*

Dealing with the etymology leads to the supposition that all rheumatic loss of articulation could, in actuality, signify an increase in constancy and steadfastness. It is as if Nature were attempting to prevent an all-too-ready, marionette-like adaptation, a tendency toward a jack-in-the-box loss of identity. Insofar as it lies within Nature's plan for joints to stiffen, chronic rheumatoid arthritis is best suited to this end. Almost nothing seems to limit mobility more effectively than *polyarthritis chronica.*

Most frequently, the disease begins insidiously between the ages of twenty and forty-five. It may have been preceded by a longer or shorter period of intense activity. The patient may have been obsessed by a compulsion for work, participation in sporting events, excessive dancing, and the like prior to the onset of the first prodromal symptoms. The disease begins in secret, as it were: now and then there is a mild fever, a feeling of malaise, weakness, and fatigue. Patients may suffer from inexplicable nervousness and irritability or experience diffuse melancholy. The developing condition may possibly be connected with local symptoms. Temporary swelling of the joints, vague discomfort in the arms and hands, and other, related symptoms appear, making a diagnostic evaluation difficult. Finally, the disease may manifest itself in stiffness and pain in the mornings, particularly in the upper extremities. Above all, the distal joints are unusually warm, swollen, and reddened. The pain extends to the musculature. Strictly symmetrical in nature, the condition travels from the peripheral, small joints to the proximal, large ones. The insidious nature of the course of the disorder mentioned in terms of time appears to repeat itself in terms of space: from the vague to the definite, from the small to the large. The disease proceeds in stages, leading to the familiar joint deformities: distention and rigidity increase as the articulated surfaces degenerate and the bones fuse ankylotically. What began as articulation terminates in a fixed structure. We are familiar with polyarthritically deformed hands: fingers like bayonets, fixed toward the ulnar face; distal joints overextended, hanging completely useless; backs of the hands sunken. Due to lack of use, the muscles around the joints atrophy, and the skin covering the joints becomes paper-thin.

The course of the disease is decidedly chronic. Deformities increase in stages although the condition can be temporarily arrested at any time. It seems almost as if Nature had intended a certain degree of deformity. Once this is attained, the pain recedes and may even totally disappear, as if the disease process possessed an intentionality, limited in time and space. In this sense, chronic polyarthritis behaves very much like the many other disorders to which mankind is subject.

Lasting over a period of decades, with increasing deformity, the disease frequently ends in death. The final phases are wretched and piteous, suited to evoke cries of protest against life's unreasonable demands. Such cries usually emanate from outsiders. Arthritics themselves are generally very patient, complain very little, and steer their way with saint-like defiance through the trials and tribulations of their lives. If we assume that Nature guards over human mortality as mercifully as she does jealously, then she has made a discovery in polyarthritis which elicits respect for her intentions which otherwise seemingly apply only to what is most deplorable in the human condition. *Belle indifference*, for example, counters the pain of the hysteric. One loses awareness of the unbearable anguish because other mechanisms are set in motion, making the condition endurable. Similarly, Nature gives arthritics their legendary indifference.

*

From the vast amount of information about the illness, we are struck by the inherent conflict between a multiform flexibility—where we hear the 'flexing' of a joint—and stoic immobility. No matter how arthritics are examined, psychologically or clinically, the same phenomenological pattern emerges. These patients seem indefatigably active; they slave overconscientiously for others; they are busy night and day on the job or at home. They remain self-effacing, forbearing to the point of submissiveness and, most of all, are without complaint.

What they lack, a kind of spontaneous 'No' toward excessive self-sacrifice, is simply expressed physically. Such patients seem to have been denied access to this 'No' as an effective, protective egotism. This lack of a natural defense appears as stiffness and deformity in the body, while the psyche remains largely unaffected. The stoic resistance materializes solely in a morphological metamorphosis, misshapen and reminiscent of crawling reptiles, a species with extremities which curiously resemble polyarthritic deformities.

Somatic blocking of jack-in-the-box submissiveness and activity is not at all specific and appears in response to a wide variety of situations. Cold, damp weather, professional and domestic factors, as well as infectious diseases and operations can contribute in equal measure to the characteristic stiffening. It is as if the flexibility of adaptation needed to take place. What was previously bearable no longer is. Electromyograms register an increase in muscle tonus to all kinds of stimuli, particularly in the areas around the affected joints. An emotionally trying interview is not the least of such stimuli. What previously would have been normal stress has become disease-producing. The stubborn defense, the somatic blocking, is capable of outlasting situations many times more demanding.

There is a belief that limiting children's motoric freedom can later lead to chronic arthritis—mothers usually being regarded as the guilty parties. This assumption is highly questionable as is the entire concept of tracing the course of disease back to early childhood. It often seems more likely that children of a particular disposition manipulate their mothers into repressive behavior. Sooner or later the pattern is repeated with others, making them into noxae, into disease-evoking factors. At a tender age their hyperactivity already constellates braking influences. This would also explain why all children in the same family, raised by the same mother, seldom contract the same disease. In the context of the origin of polyarthritis, the behavior of such mothers is readily labeled repressive and, therefore, rheumatogenic. Looked at more closely, the mother's behavior is not the actual cause, although it is symptomatic and valuable as amplification. The patient himself places no more emphasis upon this particular factor than on others which influenced the genesis of his disorder. It often seems to be our irrational need for causality which makes mothers the cause just because they are the first people who come to mind. More likely, though, it is the genetic disposition seeking from birth influences in the outside world which activates the potential into reality.

The concept that arthritis is a particularly "auto-aggressive" or self-destructive condition is also unjustified. Certainly, there is an impulse at work in arthritics, not biochemically understandable, which attempts to destroy the organism by means of infection. This impulse is in no way characteristic of rheumatoid arthritis, however, and can be found in all human illness, a death-wish programmed by Nature. It kills through infarcts, accidents, or tumors, as well as through infection. In the final analysis, human life is lived to die, preplanned suicide, a chronic death by voodoo. It is a life blessed for only a limited number of years by good health, something we do not usually appreciate.

*

Archetypal medicine would suggest that human greatness, that which comprises the 'health' or 'fitness' of mankind, could not exist without the counterpart of illness, that greatness even lives from and is driven on by disease. Basically this seems to apply to all human beings, even though the contours of uniqueness depend upon other factors as well. Stiffening of the joints, as one of our diseases, also has a counterpart of greatness. The French philosopher Emil Chartier, who is described in André Maurois's book *From Proust to Camus*, is an example.

Chartier, also an arthritic, was born in 1868 and was known by the pen-name "Alain." This unassuming pseudonym exemplifies his personality. He was not only a philosopher of patience and perseverance but also of the understatement. In him the psychosomatic characteristics of polyarthritis have found a kind of medical monument.

Chartier was not a deferential—but certainly an obedi-ent—citizen, a *citoyen contre les pouvoirs*. During World War I, at the age of forty-six, he volunteered for military service and spent the entire war as a heavy artillery gunner. He chose not to become an officer and later refused a professorial chair at the Sorbonne, remaining a high-school teacher in a French city the rest of his life. For many years, every evening without excep-tion, he wrote his famous "Propos" for a daily newspaper. He had committed himself never to write more or less than two pages, a promise he kept religiously. Chartier believed that all of his "Propos" originated because of his own free will, that they dealt with free will, and that they arose from his firm resolve to begin every morning anew. He saw these principles as the power of Man over Matter and over himself, finding therein the energy to meet the obligation for happiness.

Alain was arthritic long before he fell ill: his spirit was the spirit of the disease. For him human freedom was linked directly with morality. Despite the richness of his imagination, he was a philosopher of obedience as the foremost condition for com-munity. One hears unequivocally the polyarthritic compulsion for forbearance and the untiring dedication to duty. Maurois says that Chartier was characterized by his "vow": he felt one must commit oneself. Without commitment, ideas change from situation to situation and become no more than a passing fancy.

Although Alain wanted to be a poet, he chose to write prose instead. He found prose to be more austere, less ornamental, to be a form which forbade him from passing off lyrics as thoughts. He felt that human passions should be subjected to control and regarded the arts as the ultimate expression of such control. To discipline the emotions, to pour the body's molten protestations into molds, was true Art. In this manner, dance, song, music, and poetry came to be. The sublime is born, then, when Nature's awesomeness, its crashing thunder, and howling winds are tamed and relativized through human intellect.

In a sense, Chartier was definitely a moral philosopher. He is to be admired for a subtlety of style capable of repeatedly recasting a few basic Stoic principles in ever-new forms. However, what is most amazing is that Alain not only preached but also *practiced* what he preached. We assume that his self-discipline was an act of free will. Was this really the case? Is it not more likely that his morality arose from the motile parts of his body, from his muscles and, above all, from his joints? Was not his rigid philosophy a mouthpiece for his stiffened articulation, an inevitable conformity of mind with body?

One account observes: "His funeral at the Père-Lachaise cemetery was simple and moving."

*

Although rheumatoid arthritis exhibits the unusual quality of affecting joints symmetrically, this may vary. A thirty-five-year-old woman who was hospitalized due to an attack of arthritis in her right wrist is a case in point. Shortly after entering the clinic, she had a pathognomonic initial dream and awoke from it with her characteristic complaint:

> I'm in a large room where a large number of people are seated at tables, probably waiting for something to eat. I have to fill their glasses from heavy pitchers. It seems like I am the only one this task is entrusted to. I am being forced to do this by a man in the background who is wearing a benevolent grin. It was some kind of blackmail.

The patient awoke in the midst of the seemingly endless work and reported having pains in her wrist.

After what has already been said, it will not be especially difficult to interpret the dream. It does show how compulsive activity on behalf of others is inseparably linked to the infection and stiffening of the wrist. The dream portrays the performance of a never-ending duty as well as the serving quality which passes as altruism. At the same time, one catches a glimpse of a blackmail maneuver, of compulsions, and of a despotism which, please note, has nothing to do with the mother. The polyarthritic altruism and forbearance are clearly portrayed here as obsessions. They are seldom recognized as such and frequently occur below the threshold of consciousness.

The healthiest aspect of this patient seems to be the inflammation of her wrist, the only effective means of blocking out the unending demands placed upon her. This is particularly true considering the locus of the infection in the wrist, in the hand-joint. Her prevailing attitude was one of passivity, a "lead-me-by-the-hand" helplessness, and she would grasp at whatever or whoever was handiest to serve it.

*

Archetypal medicine's investigation of rheumatic stiffening of the joints probably leads at some point to the philosophy of the Stoics, where patience, pliancy, obedience, and altruism play significant roles. Stoicism was primarily an ethical doctrine: the effect of a way of thinking as a way of life. The purely philosophical aspects were secondary. Stoicism was a philosophy of deed, action as the measure of all wisdom, intended to make more bearable the loathsomeness of the *condition humaine* in general and in particular the mean living conditions of the Roman Empire.

At this time a number of men appeared on the scene who could best be described as "moralizers." They lived mostly in Italy and Greece but were also found in Asia Minor and Syria. They lived as simply as possible, renouncing material possessions and taking pride in bearing outer poverty with dignity. They wore only a sleeveless garment, extending barely to the knee and wrapped twice around their bodies leaving the right shoulder bare. Barefooted, carrying only a staff and knapsack, they wandered indefatigably from place to place, living from the alms of their contemporaries. Wherever they were, they discussed questions pertaining to daily life and morality. Preaching virtue, peace of mind, true freedom, and much more, they spoke about death, poverty and wealth, about honor, and against pleasures of the flesh.

They displayed defiant disdain for the body. It was filth for them by nature and for the immortal soul a cumbersome dungeon. Accordingly, they were also spartan in their nourishment: pearl barley, lupines, figs, and water were more than sufficient. They slept in temple porticos or in the baths; they bore heat and cold, hunger and thirst in almost superhuman fashion. Philosophical moderation was the order of the day and was taken for granted. Otherwise, though, one is left with a feeling of the Stoics' awkwardness toward everything and everyone. They were 'self-sufficient' and, insofar as this attitude extended to their inner lives, they were apathetic. In other words, they were untouched by their emotions, impulses, and desires.

Assuming that awkwardness and rigidity find expression as a painful stiffening of the joints the more fanatically that obedience and submission are preached, it is not surprising that one of the most famous of these moralizers, Epictetus, was rheumatic (if the account of his pupil Suidas can be believed). Epictetus was a Phrygian and lived around the middle of the first century A. D. His mother was a slave, and he himself was sold and taken early in his life to Rome where he was later set free. He was exiled to Nicopolis in Epirus during the reign of Domitian as were most of the moralizing philosophers of ancient Italy. Reading in his philosophical legacy, the *Manual* or *Encheridion*, gives the feeling of meeting one of the luminaries of the Stoic ideal. The work is a hodgepodge of unattainable demands. Assuming that there is such a thing as free will and that advice or counsel can be effective, the *Manual's* suggestions should lead to a Nirvana of honor. Human nature being what it is, however, these passages from Epictetus seem sanctimonious and owe their lofty one-sidedness to the support of a solid, bony shadow. Unless it is directed specifically at rheumatics, does the following advice have any real value?

> This wretched body does not concern me! Its limbs do not concern me! Death? Let it come when it will, be it for all mankind, be it for only one among us! [or] Look at me! I have no fatherland, no

home, neither property nor servants. I sleep on the bare earth. . . . yet, have I worries? or fear? Am I not truly free? When has one of you seen that I desired something and did not obtain it? avoided something and still succumbed to it? . . .

Human fantasy seems to rise from the same depths as human illness. These are areas far beyond the limits of consciousness where phenomena originate according to fixed principles. Only in retrospect can we realize or even surmise their connection to the depths, to the abyss of our being. One might, therefore, consider whether objects of human adornment are not one of these phenomena from the 'depths.' Might not ornaments which are worn as bracelets, bangles, and rings be a symbolic representation of the relationship between articulation and rigidity?

Adorning the jointed areas—wrists, ankles, and neck—is probably a universal custom since there is hardly a culture where it is not practiced. It continues to play an important role even among the most scantily-clad tribes. It is difficult for one to relegate the phenomenon to the realm of coincidental aesthetics as the ethnologists do. Instead, one feels compelled to place these creations, equally bizarre and artistic, in a more profound context.

Certainly this particular form of adornment hints at shackles, at being bound or confined. There is a parallel to the well-worn image of the prisoner dragging a massive ball and chain behind him. The prisoner's 'hands are tied,' at the wrist actually, at that point where the hand, the specifically human instrument of action, is joined to the rest of the body. Although we speak of being bound 'hand and foot,' we usually mean the wrists and the ankles.

It would be unforgivably one-sided, however, to interpret ornamentation of the jointed areas as a pejoratively intended limitation of one's freedom of motion. Ornamentation alludes just as clearly to the need for necessary restraint, for 're-serve,' to the need for control over obedient flexibility. It is as if man were aware of the joints' unruly tendencies and adorned them as a reminder and a caveat. Adornment then serves as an apotropaic measure against rheumatic stiffness, as if man sought to forestall stiffening through a continual reminder of its existence. There is little doubt that the copper and zinc rings worn as a protection against rheumatism owe their existence to such transcendental associations.

Joint ornamentation is seldom plain. On the contrary, unusual amounts of time and money are spent on it in addition to the high level of manual dexterity and artistic ability necessary for its production. Considering that what is created serves as a substitute for rheumatism, the process is almost reminiscent of an alchemical opus. It is as if man sought to illuminate the gold in the depths of the existential horror which is paralysis and deformity. It is as if he sought to create symbols in which uninhibited exuberance and necessary restraint come together.

On Pain and Punishment

BASED on its physiology, pain results from excesses, from damage to the body exceeding normal wear and tear which sets in where the contact of blow, bite, break, or cut was destructive. Pain comes from excessive stretching or straining or the application of pressure. It occurs when overheating or undercooling exceeds a particular limit. It can be the result of chemical compounds, gastric juices, for example, which when produced in excess affect the lining of the gastrointestinal tract. Pain occurs around the infected areas if the tissue has been disturbed beyond a certain point. Above all, pain results when all of the above-mentioned trauma take place at a certain minimal rate of speed.

Physiologically, pain sets in when the damaged tissue secretes substances, metabolic noxae, which emit a sufficient impulse for pain or 'damage' to be registered. These substances are the polypeptides, proteins which originate in the blood plasma: serotonin, histamine, and hydrogen and potassium ions. Inasmuch as they all stimulate peripheral pain perception, they are all capable of evoking what is referred to as 'pain.' The stimulus is then sent to the brain over a network serving that particular purpose and comprised of nerve cells with either thick, rapidly-conducting fibers or long, slowly-conducting fibers. The nerves pass through the posterior stem into the spinal cord and conduct the pain via the anterior column of the spinal cord to the thalamus, which in turn is connected to the cortex of the parietal lobe.

When speaking of pain, we differentiate between light or surface pain and the dull, protopathic pain which originates deep
within the tissues. Surface pain is registered in the upper dermal
layers from pinpricks, pinches, and the like and carries little
significance for a consideration of the principals of the pain
phenomenon. It is sometimes related to itching, to *pruritus*, and
results in numerous defensive and avoidance reactions. The
deeper, protopathic pain can stem from all of the injuries mentioned at the beginning. It may arise from the musculature, the
bones and tendons, from the joints, the arterial walls, the
mucous linings, the intestines, or from the musculature of
tubular organs such as the renal pelvis or uterus. It is especially
'emotional' in nature, affecting us totally due to its indeterminate origin and its tendency to radiate into surrounding
areas. Avoidance or resistance occurs very seldom with protopathic pain: we tend to remain as quiet as possible, hardly
daring to move or, at most, turning from side to side. Generally,
nonetheless, we are wide awake, pulse and blood pressure are increased, as if we were extremely alarmed or were performing an
exceedingly strenuous task.

*

Someone suffering from migraine headaches hides himself
away in a darkened room, groaning between changes of cold
compresses. Someone afflicted with a gallstone or kidney-stone
attack fidgets and complains. The patient who feels as if pain
had a stranglehold on his heart silently clenches his teeth, while
the one with hemorrhoids doubles over in agony. None of them
seem able to move, as if they had been nailed to the spot or
gripped by an invisible hand.

From the perspective of archetypal medicine, these various
forms of martyrdom belong to that chimerical tendency in man
which mediates participation in the paradoxes of pain and
pleasure. It is as if the degeneration of illness were the physical
form taken by a "hurting-myself-and-others" transformed into

pain to be realized and recognized. It seems as if pain were the only way torment and pleasure are released from chaotic entanglement with one another to assert their separate and independent existences. It is as if some kind of sadistic dowry, denied its rightful place in individual lives and caught in hesitation, found its way into the body without detracting from existing scruples and amiability. In point of fact, psychosomatic medicine believes that all forms of malaise accompanied by pain are often but the various forms assumed by hostility as it poaches whatever attention it can. This holds true for headaches, gall and kidney stones, angina pectoris, the pain of hemorrhoids, rheumatic suffering, the aches of fractures, and much more.

These forms of aggression rage in the body as pain but are not really 'animal' in nature, rather tortures peculiar to man. Animals seem to hate and suffer differently, more 'naturally,' which may explain science's use of laboratory animals and the tortures to which they are subjected. Perhaps science rightly assumes that animals experience pain differently from human beings, that animal pain lacks an intellectual/satanic element. By contrast, human beings are not only animals which can say "no," as Nietzsche would have it, but are also animals capable of torturing in a unique way. This characteristic stood man in good stead as he set about building his own world and contributed greatly to the survival of the species homo sapiens. The specific quality of human pain may reside in the fact that man's capacity for dealing out pain also exhibits especially satanic characteristics. Accordingly, *human pain would be sadism in physical, corporeal form* which for one reason or another we are incapable of dealing with.

*

In the view of archetypal medicine, human abilities and talents tend to become destructive when they succumb to the tendency to become absolutes, to lead astray, or to be elevated to the position of ideals. At such times Nature makes the necessary correction on the physical plane, especially when the normal psychopathic adversities at her disposal fail to bring about the desired effect. Nature's correction counterbalances elements of human society with a corresponding illness, at least to the extent that such social forms become too one-sidedly directed toward justice, peace, or kindness or become too agreeable, too proper, or too respectable. Nature seems to have a rather morbid fantasy in such matters and possesses an extensive arsenal of possibilities in terms of physical suffering with which she manifests various forms of antisocial aggressivity. The utopia of "peaceful coexistence," what might be termed "social pleasure" and a generalized altruism, demands a price which cannot be paid simply in the currency of 'psychic' disturbances. In addition, each variety of social utopia attracts a corresponding form of suffering, and it is inevitable that our modern, social ideal is linked to the very diseases which make up our contemporary epidemics.

Much that is antisocial finds expression as physical pain and, in this larval form, populates our hospitals and nursing homes. The remainder, in the form of criminality, reverts to the judicial system which, from the standpoint of archetypal medicine, can be viewed as an institution for the artificial administration of pain. When human aggression does not become mired in its own swamp or become cushioned by rather questionable diseases, jurisprudence hands down a prison sentence which tortures and which is intended to torture. Its purpose is to make the individual in question dis-eased, sick!

Here, in the realm of the penal code, is where man's satanical qualities have borne the motliest assortment of fruit: criminals have been decapitated, scourged, stoned, and beaten. Noses and ears have been cut off, to say nothing of genitals; offenders have been broken on the wheel, impaled, and quartered, have been ground to death, hanged, singed, burned at the stake, and blinded. In the name of justice, human beings have been put in chains or made to pull millstones and, occasionally, have been disemboweled. There appears to be no kind of pain which has not at one time or another been included in the repertory of one penal code or another, including the immobilizing experience of the sickbed which jurisprudence reproduced in the rack. Inflicting physical pain was only so popular because it was the most practical. It is much easier to torture a delinquent physically than it is to induce an asthmatic attack, for example, although burning at the stake has something in common with asthma inasmuch as victims of both die from suffocation.

The forms of punishment have varied with the times. The punishment meted out today by the courts is how we moderns make someone sick because of his antisocial hostilities. The basic principle, though, has remained the same: plus ca change, mais plus c'est la meme chose. Our courts impose deprivation and frustration by placing criminals in prison or by levying fines: both the loss of freedom and loss of property are effective to the extent that such measures inflict physical or quasi-physical pain. There is a profusion of unpleasant, endosomatic sensations which give the modern penal code its real value. It is completely conceivable that a later age will discover other ways of administering 'artificial' pain in the service of the concept of a just and peaceful society.

*

When we investigate etymologically the terms of pain, we discover that one of the closest linguistic relatives of "pain" is "punishment," as if pain and punishment were linked at the deepest levels in the origins of human speech. The Indo-Germanic root (s)merd meant merely 'to chafe,' in the sense of 'to scrub' or 'to be chafed.' It reoccurs in Greek as smerdnos 'ghastly' or in the Latvian merdet 'emaciate.' The connection between pain and punishment is more apparent in the etymol-

ogy of the German *Weh* 'pain,' which was originally an urlaut.*
Its Indo-Germanic root is *uai* which appears in Latin as *vae!*
'woe,' in the phrase *vae victis!* ("woe to the conquered!"), and in
the German *weinen* 'to cry,' probably originally 'to sob for woe.'
The relationship between pain and punishment seen in connection with the word "woe" (German *Weh*) is also found with
"pain" or, in the German, *Pein.* "Pain" traces its etymological
genealogy to the Latin *poena* 'punishment,' the middle Latin
pena 'torment of hell,' and the Greek *poine*, which means
'penance.' Small wonder that in earlier times the hangman was
somewhat sadistically called, in German, *Peinlein* 'little pain'!

The patient was a kindly, somewhat overly polite accountant
who had spent his life in straitened circumstances and amidst
doubts and scruples. Always rather anxious and hypochon-
driac, he led a Walter Mitty existence punctuated by erotic, but
sexually abortive, escapades. He tended to be flighty and superficial and occasionally even extravagant. The 'pleasures of the
world' had always been a source of temptation and anxiety for
him. Even if he did demonstrate a certain aversion for work, it
was never severe enough to cause him to lose his job.

For decades he maintained a tenuous balance between fickle-
ness and barely sufficient self-discipline until, at the age of fifty,
he was struck with utter devastation. He became his own ac-
cuser: he confessed his escapades to his wife, for she had become
his moral conscience. She had always advised and controlled
him, had sacrificed herself for his sake, and had filled their common existence with burdensome seriousness. She had led the
respectable life of a kind of martyr, becoming prematurely gray.
She had always been trustworthy for him, because her good intentions seemed unsullied by any of his doubts. His confession
awakened accusations, confusion, sympathy, and hatred in his
wife, and he persecuted himself with sadistic fantasies. He imagined throwing himself in front of a train and being cut to

* Combined form from the German *ur* 'primeval,' 'original' and the German
laut 'sound,' 'tone.'

pieces, being buried by a stream of onrushing automobiles, or standing homeless on the street, impoverished and wasted in body and mind. In his self-torment, he reproached himself for the dissoluteness of his past and repressed any inspirations to the contrary.

Religion became a trial for him: his spiritual and psychic life consisted almost entirely of self-accusations, degenerating into a hellish purgatory of greed for punishment and the torment of guilt feelings. In a manner of speaking, he chastised himself. He refused all antidepressive medication and tranquilizers, leaving them untouched or taking them in such small doses they had no effect. If someone insisted that he take medication and administered it to him, an unpredictable, negative placebo reaction set in, and his condition only deteriorated more.

In addition to the deplorable psychic changes which took place in the patient, there was a profusion of physical tortures: his gastrointestinal tract was particularly affected, especially the colon, the anus, and the pelvic floor. His mouth was dry, and he continually felt like retching or throwing up. In a very short time he had lost forty-five pounds. He was also plagued by constipation, painful hemorrhoids, and anal cramping originating deep under the coccyx. He complained that the lower part of his body was "deaf," that his genitals were "dead," and that sort of thing. He was impotent and regarded it as the expression of an obstinate defiance. Although his internist prescribed a number of appropriate medications, he refused to make regular use of them since he felt that he was not deserving of them.

His medical condition was associated with a tendency toward superstitious interpretations of daily banalities. He wouldn't dare, for example, write letters with black ink out of fear they would harm whoever received them. He thought that he came from Russia (in German, *Russland*, literally 'soot land'), from a country where everything was black and gray. His sadistically distorted view of the world extended to his dreams as well: once he dreamed of a dark, dragon-like, and revolting animal with a mouth filled with small, pointed teeth which chewed up a piglet. Even though the dreamer wanted to protest, someone advised him against it. In fact the patient seemed possessed by an archaic compulsion for destruction and revenge, by powers characterized in antiquity as sauropodic pythons and by Christianity as animal avatars of the devil. In the above dream, they appear as exaggerated pangs (is there not an onomatopoeic connection here to "pain"?) of conscience, as if the patient's innocent 'piggishness' had become grist for the mill of his conscience. Recognizing the facts of his situation was of little help to him. He spent many years in a psychiatric clinic and was finally declared to be a chronic case.

*

Somatization may be understood as a form of compensation which most inconsiderately compels us to rectify an exaggeratedly one-sided relationship to our environment. How we regard this compensatory quality depends on our predisposition: we perceive it either as a moral issue or as an experience full of mystic awe. The pious tend to see somatization as punishment for a life of sin, interpreting the experience within the framework of an authoritarian Deity who 'visits' his wrath upon the errant. This view prevails in religious traditions other than the Judaeo-Christian: Zeus and Allah carry out their 'visitations' as well. To what extent the concept of visitation and punishment has meaning depends in large measure upon the individual and the prevailing collective typology. When an undue emphasis upon self-denial and utopian fantasies of peaceful coexistence evokes the somatization of a natural sadism, one is certainly entitled to speak of 'punishment.'

Somatization appears less as chastisement by a divine Being for those who tend toward mystic awe or who harbor a propensity for 'natural law,' for those characterized by a sense of polarities and proportions and for whom ecology takes precedence over morals. They would perceive in somatization the workings of the greater wisdom and the numinosity of the laws of nature. Such was the case for Carl von Linné, Carolus Linnaeus, who developed our system for plant classification in his work *Systema Naturae*. In Linnaeus's mind, the concept of world order as maintained by a God of judgment changed to one of an order determined by a *nemesis divina*. In his book with the same title, he discusses the Old Testament idea of retribution as a kind of natural, ecological happening, adding in a commentary that he himself had peeked over God's shoulder. Linnaeus belongs within the Swedish tradition which began with Emanuel Swedenborg's *Oeconomia Regni Naturae*, a tradition which mediated between scientific/empirical thinking and religious belief. There are also parallels to August Strindberg whose writings during the 1890s were heavily influenced by the spirit of "romantic chemistry." With his concept of a *nemesis divina*, though, Linnaeus also belongs in a very general way to the tradition of Theodosius and especially to that of physico-theology. The latter is a skeptical doctrine of proportions introduced by William Derham concerning the divine equilibrium of the world.

We cannot overlook the fact that the philosophical ideas of the Marquis de Sade also lie within the perspective of physico-theology. 'Sadism' consists of more than simply tidbits of perversity, being the complete Weltanschauung of a libertine, an aristocratic ethic in which the spreading of pain and suffering belongs to one's daily tasks. Sade protested against the reign of terror of Christian charity. He propagated a countermorality which, at the same time, he incorporated in a more comprehensive ethical theory, and he became an apologist for crime as part of natural, social order. In this sense he is very much related philosophically to Swedenborg, Derham, Linnaeus, and Strindberg. He did, however, exceed the others in audacity, a trait which almost cost him his life. All of these thinkers seem to be characterized by a kind of melancholic stoicism or cynicism.

*

In the fifteenth century, Hieronymus Bosch painted a gigantic triptych including scenes entitled "Garden of Delight" and "Hell," which have served Christian orthodoxy for centuries as allegorical representations for wantonness and its hellish consequences. Contemporaries have occasionally voiced the opinion that the work was intended to be the altarpiece for a sect outside the Church, for some group of mystics who never made a name for themselves and have left no record of their existence.

The thoughts and images that must have gone through Bosch's mind approach the concepts of archetypal medicine. Bosch seems, with his prolific fantasy and love for detail, to have been attempting to portray how exaggerated health leads or yields to disease. In particular, he seems to show how love of one's fellow man, how gregarious pleasures intended to bring about the perfection of a paradise on earth, gives way to sadism and pain. The portion of the triptych labeled "Garden of Delight" can well be regarded as a social paradise. It is not difficult to recognize motifs and themes that are cultivated when the desire for peaceful coexistence is of primary importance. As has been the case in historical models of social utopias, the motifs seem somehow exaggerated. Bosch wants to make it clear that before one gets to "Hell" one has first to experience a form of self-seduction, the unreality of collective bliss or a kind of hubris of caritas.

Although the painting is overpopulated with naked bodies, nowhere are there tumults or riots to be seen. On the contrary, everywhere there are gentle, peaceful groupings of people who are apparently happy and mutually considerate. Despite the happiness, though, there is a sense of agitation, of unrest, willfulness, and emptiness. In one place men go galloping off on stags, horses, pigs, bears, and cattle in snappy formations, giving the feeling of a cavalry-like discipline or the regulation of modern automobile traffic. All the while the riders cannot help but perform reckless acrobatics, contortions which on a running animal must surely end in disaster. And yet, there is no sign at all of any such painful accidents!

The women and maidens are likewise assembled here and there in groups and clusters. They tend more to put their heads together, to play and splash in charming pools, and to balance fruit and birds on their heads. They enjoy dancing, even the apostate nuns among them who still wear veils, albeit transparent ones, on their half-shorn heads. Of course, there is no discrimination here: Moorish women are included in the groups. The community and solidarity of all human beings is the order of the day, even if there are so many human beings that the paradise of Nature is on the brink of being trampled underfoot.

In Bosch's rendition, there are only naked beings in the "Garden of Delight." Gone is the Gregorian phobia of nakedness, and mutual trust is not only spiritual but physical as well. People can be close to one another without guile: embraces are tender, kisses delicate. Even anality has its totally wondrous significance: dainty flowers grow out of or are placed in the anal opening. In the Garden of Delight there is no hostility, hate, or torment. It is as if Satan had never been heard of—but also as if something were missing and as if some unperceived storm must be brewing over so much joy in one place.

There seem to be no worries either about what to do for food: the juicy fruit and sparkling berries produced by the luxuriant flora are used mostly for play. And the fruit is amazing! It glistens and flashes like gemstones, making the very sight of it a tactile experience. The naked populace carries it around, grinning and playing ball with it, apparently one of the primary activities. On the whole, the people give the impression of comprising *the* affluent society, a "no-deposit-no-return" attitude of unconscious exploitation.

It comes as no surprise that this social paradise is also primarily an aesthetic landscape where one has difficulty determining where nature stops and where the inventions of man's sense of art begin. The painting seems to have captured what modern science is striving toward: technical beauty for everyone. A fountain of life stands in one of the pools, but is it a rare form of plant-life or an inorganic piece of sculpted art made of glass and gems? Wondrous balls of glass give way to stone as if nothing were more natural, and the human beings find hiding places in the curious rock formations as if no more enchanting kind of security existed.

*

Since all forms of pain and sadism are missing in "Garden of Delight," it will come as no surprise that Bosch's vision of Hell is correspondingly revolting. Bosch's inferno is as much a place of diabolical suffering as the first panel is one of pure enjoyment. Bosch seems to adhere to almost mathematical standards for pain and pleasure in his images of social utopia and catastrophe. One should bear in mind that neither Heaven nor Hell is limited in its significance to the moral/theological, but both are also areas of pathology. Hell is not merely a place defined by various religions as penance, hellfire, or eternal damnation but also one of the purest images of human illness.

Even though human beings are to some extent aware of their own guilt—theologically, their own sin—by and large they perceive themselves free from both, guilt and sin. They act like most patients act: as if their diseases were trials or afflictions beyond their control and their aetiological comprehension. In Bosch's inferno they are surprised in their state of innocence or, in contemporary psychological terms, in their state of unconsciousness. They have no idea where all the pain they are suffering has come from, just as they have no realization of the absurd lengths to which they go in the name of health. They remain blissfully unaware of the extent of their pathogenic attitudes and behavior.

Whereas a freshness and coolness predominated in the Garden of Delight and a pastel light gave the landscape an ethereal quality, Hell is bathed in shades of scarlet and subjected to lethal heat emanating from a burning city cast against a night sky. Whereas paradise was filled with the most subtle and delicate fragrances, one can almost smell the smoke of the inferno, while the chorus of birdsong has given way to a terrifying cacophony of moaning and howling from trumpets, trombones, kettle drums, and bagpipes. Where pleasure was evident before in the relaxed and unencumbered mobility, now in Hell people are bound, muzzled, and nailed down in positions which, without exception, are inescapably agonizing.

Even nakedness assumes a different character. Where in paradise it was related to trust and mutual goodwill, in Hell it becomes the carrier of human vulnerability and the unprotectedness of man's insufficient nature. Happiness is gone from the faces. Now one sees looks of horror, surprise, anxiety, or the distortion of pain. Where the Garden of Delight was filled with spontaneously formed groups, Hell reveals a splintering-off into isolation, into the loneliness only experienced by one in pain.

What is overly healthy reverts to its opposite, to what is sick. Delight reverses into pain. A jagged knife-blade is drawn across a sufferer's back; another person is spread-eagled on a harp, subjected like one tortured on a wheel to fractures and dislocations. Gluttony, in the form of snapping dogs, assaults one defenseless soul, while a second holds his ears lest his head burst from the thundering drone. Here a victim is stabbed; there a jaundiced figure vomits. Even anality has shifted position: where previously flowers grew out of the anus, now there is a gigantic bassoon instead, entering the anus to reemerge above the shoulders and forcing the poor victim to walk all bent over. Out of other anal openings black birds escape or flatuses pipe grotesquely on flutes!

If archetypal medicine views human pain as being woven into the interplay of love and hate as a physical manifestation of hate, Bosch's triptych could express this concept. Archetypal medicine also sees the pathogenic effect of an undue emphasis on human 'health,' sees how recessive characteristics still manage to assert themselves and, like the painter of the Middle Ages, sees how human life always has a distinctly negative prognosis. In the light of this prognosis, Bosch, like archetypal medicine, would both hold man responsible and exonerate him only to a certain extent. On the one hand, there is too much innocence and naïvete written on the faces of Bosch's characters for them to know really what is happening to them. On the other hand, their behavior is too frivolous for him to absolve them of all responsibility.

For Bosch, as well, discernment seems to serve as a means of diluting and sublimating an all-too-painful reality. It is as if he, too, like his characters, were incapable of actually experiencing the full reality of the situation. In his triptych, everything seems to be presented only in its essence and, despite the extensive use of details, is symbolical—even allegorical—in style. The result is an alienation, a certain anaesthetization, a reassuring super-elevation of the importune, and a distancing from everything that would come too close. Can this way of experiencing be seen as similar to the area of prepsychotic dreariness, a lack of direct emotion which is schizoid or ironically puerile in nature? The question is not so farfetched when one considers that much of the art of the Middle Ages was done within this perspective or Weltanschauung. Everything is seen from the point of view of the eternal and therefore carries a sense of fruitlessness, temporality, of being just a passing fancy. The ephemeral character is only further emphasized by the portrayal of immense spaces, overwhelming panoramas, and the use of an irrational perspective. The end effect is a strange resonance as from heavenly choirs, as if an otherworldly music became audible amidst the everyday occurrences portrayed with such detailed pedantry. It seems that Bosch and the Middle Ages in general were capable of bringing reassurance to the realism of human existence by the presentation of the concretely material in idealized, ethereal, and highly symbolical fashion.

Just as with Bosch, archetypal medicine also considers the releasing effect of the symbolical to be of central importance. Archetypal medicine also reflects an attitude of dualistic and polar extremes in their pure forms. Despite the fact that archetypal medicine also does not lose sight of the mortal quality of human existence, it is less pessimistic than the picture we have from Bosch of the Middle Ages' view of life. Archetypal medicine looks to idealization for purposes of a therapeutic effect, not only as a gentle consolation for the fact that we must exist. In addition to the one-way street to death of human life, archetypal medicine sees much which can be reversed; it is not that health and suffering are so absolute in their separation as in the Middle Ages but that they are more intertwined.

*

Mankind possesses a deep longing for the Kingdom of God, a longing which manages to support the belief that such a thing, at some time, at some place, will become reality. In this heavenly Jerusalem there will be no pain and no sadism: there the lamb lies down with the lion, beauty reigns everywhere, and the air is filled with pleasant fragrances and heavenly harmony. The notion is so widespread among the various races and cultures and has existed in so many eras of human history that one is forced to assume that it is an integral part of human nature. The Kingdom of God is certainly possible, even if it is generally a temporary and incomplete psychic condition, experienced as absolute only in visions.

By comparison, mankind has tended to combine everything painful and sadistic under the rubric of Hell, a notion equally as ubiquitous as the Kingdom of God. Here is where all the tortures and evil of which man is capable are collected together. Here dissension dominates in all quarters, and the hateful, the perverse, and the distorted reign. Here is the stench of sulfur and other unbearable, penetrating odors and, in place of harmonic tones, dissonant cacophonies. While the redeemed often move or fly freely in a three-dimensional heavenly expanse, the damned suffer their pains in hellish torture chambers. But our hells, as well, are not just somewhere and sometime: they are much more a part of human nature itself; they are very real and immediate conditions. Just as a longing creates a Kingdom of God, so a Hell is created with an equal degree of necessity. It seems as if there were some imbedded urge attracting us, a bottomless fascination emitted by those hells of ours, as if we found it unbearable to have to live in a condition of divine wholeness and health. Human pride and self-esteem seem to require a primeval mistrust as well, a hate of creation; they seem to require the cultivation of an annihilating "No" and the desire to be suffering and sick.

Satan, the central figure of all hells, is a devilish being who often gives the impression of being severely ill when his luciferian, diabolical intelligence is overlooked. "Der Geist, der stets verneint"—Faust's "spirit of continual negation"—often ails with a curious pallor, a cyanotic gray, or a fire-black. Emaciated in face and body, he is often wasted away to nothing but skin and bones. Satan's general negativism and disdain for everything which God has created combines with a physical marasmus. He is in pain. At best, he is ill-humored, peevish, and rebuffing. Gloom stares out of the deep sadness of his eyes. His pre-psychotic, lonely melancholy is lasting and irrevocable. While one can only imagine the Christian God as hale and hearty, Satan is often chronically incurable and invalided, the counterpart for all eternity of that God for whom cherubs raise their hosannas. Just as Hell and the Kingdom of Heaven are human conditions, so too is Satan a human characteristic, the purest product of fantasy or, rather, an attitude and, as such, not something we meet in everyday reality. As least as far as pain and sadism are concerned, his is the form or the personification of the repressed aspects of God, the complete shadow figure. He would be the pain and evil of God, qualities which we never meet en masse but in thousands of 'diluted' forms at every turn.

Just as there is a liturgy to the honor of God, there were cults to the honor of Satan, although, as heresies, their activities had to take place in secret. To culminate their services of worship, cult members gave Satan a kiss, usually on the anus. It was not so much that the anus was the only place which could or should be kissed but that it was the part of the body which made Satan one of the suffering: he was possessed of his pain. Of course, this was all blasphemy as far as the official doctrine of the Church was concerned, and if participation in a Satan's mass could be proven, the offender would surely be burned at the stake. In principle, the Church acted no differently than modern medicine does in its attempt to eradicate everything perceived as not belonging. Like the Inquisition, medicine employs all sorts of chicanery to achieve this goal.

The kissing of a diseased or painful part of the body, though, is by no means a practice limited to satanic cults. It is very much a therapeutic measure in all kinds of paramedical practices like the laying-on of hands or the actual licking with the tongue of infected parts of the anatomy. A certain pathophilia is involved in these practices, an inclination bordering on the perverse toward everything sick and painful. Bearing this in mind, one is tempted to regard the satanic cults in a very different light. The so-called heretics must have been privy to a knowledge carried by a deeper, psychosomatic awareness, namely, that Satan was a poor unfortunate who was forced to assume the role of God's counterpart and became sick as a result. The kiss of the serpent, then, was a redemptive attempt to transform satanic sadisms manifested as bodily pain. When there is no respect, even love, for satanic phenomena as they are, they remain as importunate as visions of the Kingdom of God remain fictitious.

In this sense, there is a basic kinship between the cults of Satan and archetypal medicine. Archetypal medicine, too, is 'unofficial.' Archetypal medicine, too, has a tendency to defend what is most maligned and, by confirmation, releases it from somatic entanglement.

Medicine as an empirical science is as consistent in its endeavor to eradicate illness as the church is in its struggle with evil,

Fever

IN a world where we no longer produce enough emotional warmth, where we are overcome by chills and seized by fever, medical folklore finds images that have reappeared for centuries. They always revolve around an atmosphere of dread, of things dead and lifeless, cold or cool—perhaps a landscape in late autumn, in late winter, or perhaps a human scenery. These images evoke memories of dreadful weather and of experiences when we were overcome with horror, like the notion that fever is caused by a white mouse crawling out from under cold, gray stones in order to slip into the human body. Fever's imagery includes all those women and maidens who, with euphemistic or infantile-sadistic intentions, have been named *Rüddele* or *Rüddelweibchen*—'little shakers' or 'little shaking women'—creatures of a white or gray color who enter the human body and shake it in the chills of fever. Uncanny, too, is the lonely ghost that rides on a gray horse through the country in order to take possession of its inhabitants.

Goethe has captured such powerfully expressive images in his poem "Der Erlkönig," in which the elf-king seizes upon a child whom a peasant is cradling in his arms as he rides through night and wind to his farm. A whole fever-producing phantasmagoria is built up here as an illusive reinterpretation of objects that are quite natural at other times. The threatening and seductive voice of the age-old elf-king is actually the frosty rustling of the wind in the trees; his silvery-cold long hair and his white, fluttering garments are really streaks of an autumnal mist. His dangerous daughters, whom the child sees drifting through the air, are the misinterpreted shapes of old gray willows by the stream. The child dies before the father reaches the farm—in a *status febrilis*, as we would say today, of unknown aetiology.

Depending on the phase of the fever process, medical folklore has invented treatment practices which are still used to some extent, though in different forms. One of these treatments was to have the patient sleep in a baking oven while it was still warm: the fact that the oven or the hearth was always the focal point of the home—and as such diffused emotional warmth—was probably as important as the actual supply of physical warmth. Today we cover the fever patient with warm blankets, we let him perspire and fuss about him with all kinds of trifles that often warm more symbolically than physically. Folk healers also worked frequently with the blood and sweat of the sick person. With his own blood, for example, the patient would write his name on a piece of paper and then eat it. The purpose of such *Fresszettel* 'eating papers' was to consume that which was diseased in the patient's body in order to integrate it more fully. He consequently pursued a sort of auto-immunization.

*

As is well-known, man is one of the warm-blooded creatures, an organism that can maintain its body temperature within a relatively narrow range. This phenomenon, among many others, indicates the fact that all of man's dependences on the outer world are only relative. Experience shows that his constitution provides not only the conservation of necessary heat but also the maintenance of life's many other inner conditions—not the least of which are emotions such as anxiety, hostility, and guilt. These emotions arise not only from the environment but also from within, endogenously, as our dreams prove most distinctly. Thus a definite, though often puzzling, program of homeostasis, of equilibrium, is pursued.

Homoiothermia refers to the temperature prevalent in the body's core. Peripheral areas of the body, however, behave in the *poikilothermic* manner of cold-blooded creatures: that is, by varying their warmth to some extent according to outside conditions. Rectal temperature will give us the most exact information about the situation in the core, while oral and axillary temperatures will be always somewhat lower.

The conservation of a generally constant body temperature presupposes a series of nervous structures and hormonal mechanisms, of which those in the brain stem play a decisive role. The integration centers of heat regulation are accommodated in the hypothalamic area of the diencephalon; indeed, it seems as if its upper regions can bring about a cooling and its lower regions a warming effect, a discovery which resulted from the destruction of these respective areas. Besides the hypothalamus, however, the *formatio reticularis*, with its features for stimulation control, and a whole series of higher and lower segments of the nervous system also participate in regulating the body's temperature. Constant provisions are made for a small amount of heat generation that continues even during periods of rest or of external heat. This minimal production of warmth is called basal metabolism.

To ensure this regulation, temperature sensors are needed as well as efferent fibers on which the innervating impulses for appropriate measures in the body can proceed. Such sensors are situated in the diencephalon itself and in the skin. Apparently, diencephalon sensors react especially to a possible overheating, while skin receptors react mainly to a possible supercooling. The countermeasures consist either in a variable heat generation or else in a variable heat emanation. On the one hand heat generation, experienced as a sensation of freezing and shivering in the muscular system, occurs chemically by means of combustion processes in the liver and other inner organs. Heat emanation, on the other hand, is accomplished by dilated capillaries which let more blood flow to the body's surface and thereby permit increased radiation and conduction of heat. In addition, there is evaporation of moisture through the skin or through the sweat glands.

Usually we become accustomed to a certain outside temperature 'centrally,' endogenously. Thus it is not the temperature
sensors in the periphery which grow tired during continuous
cold; rather we adjust ourselves internally. We adapt ourselves
so that cold is perceived as relative warmth and, conversely,
warmth as relative cold. It is as if our 'frustration tolerances' or,
respectively, 'indulgence tolerances' were changing, and such
changes describe the phenomenon mentioned earlier: namely,
that the human constitution is capable of creating the inner
climate necessary for its own life, and that homoiothermia is a
part of this process.

*

Now every understanding of fever is determined by the
regulated connection between cold and heat. Without a consideration of this relationship, all reflections about febrility
seem to run into an impassable dead end: as, for example, when
fever is regarded as an expression or a somatic equivalent for
anxiety. In this way we would have to consider most of the
pathological cases that occupy psychosomatic medicine as an
'expression' of anxiety, whether it be a respiratory disorder, a
diarrhea, or something else. On the contrary, wherever we look,
an intertwining of cold and heat is evident in fever.[1] In this way
it behaves no differently from many other syndromes: if we attempt to comprehend asthmatic complaints, we find a combina-
tion of expiratory violence and a feeling of suffocation; in an
itching skin irritation, indolence is mixed with the rush of enthusiasm; in diarrhea, parsimony is mingled with generosity;
and in urinary disorders, decorum with heresy.

In observing the course of an ordinary fever, we already encounter this reciprocal interdependency of cold and heat. It
begins with freezing and chills, with shivering and chattering of
teeth. At the same time, the temperature usually climbs to a
high point and descends with sensations of heat—or, said
physiologically, under increased emanation of heat. The skin

which before was white, dry, and cool reddens and is covered with perspiration.

The beginning of a fever, like the adaptation to a new thermic climate, is also centrally regulated; the organism adjusts itself. This so-called *Sollverstellung*—'adjustment of the normal condition'—is a change of disposition, as it were, so that an external temperature that previously seemed neutral or even warm is now perceived as cold, and the system is forced to heat itself. This remarkable inner adaptation can be understood not only physically but psychically as well; it may happen when not only physical cold but also a mental atmosphere of chronic coolness and distance is no longer endurable. It may also take place under the image of 'impaired resistance' when the frustration tolerance weakens. All feelings of emptiness and of being misunderstood, of nervous impatience, and many others can be obviated by a somatic overheating—that is, by fever. The subsistence of psychic heat generation in the substance of the body is the essence of the process called fever.

When, therefore, psychosomatic authors regard febrility as an expression of anxiety, this anxiety is rather a chill which does not quite enter one's consciousness; the fever suddenly, for example, occurring in toddlers or school children, at the first day of a new employment, or during the honeymoon is less anxiety than an irremovable chill. This holds true not only for those 'psychogenic' febrile conditions that can be qualified by few somatic symptoms but also for many physical diseases as, for instance, influenza infections and other ailments whose leading symptom is fever.

Thus febrility behaves in essentially the same way as all other syndromes which can become manifest 'psychogenically' as well as 'somatogenically'; its nature remains the same in both cases. Consequently, we find in ordinary headaches similar regularities as in migraine; in colitis serosa or ulcerosa similar patterns as in infectious diarrhea; in nervous angina pectoris as in cardiac infarction; or in blushing as in dermatoses concomitant to erythema. The nature of fever does not seem to be governed only by these so-called diseases; it rather takes on variable degrees of somatization and in this respect behaves similarly to the syndromes mentioned above, which are distinguished by their varying degrees of materialization.

Fever is a necessary condition—*not-wendig* in German: 'need-averting'—that makes use of 'reasons': for example, of 'essential mechanisms' or of bacteria and virus which it compels to become virulent. Of course, such a view of feverish diseases is rather obsolete in contemporary medicine, especially since it reminds us of a time when symptoms and syndromes *were* 'the diseases,' when there was "the hot and the cold burn" (erysipelas and gangrene), and when physicians rarely understood diseases from aetiological points of view. Nevertheless an old nosology, guided by symptoms, is more natural to a psychosomatic, 'archetypal' medicine than to a modern one; symptoms like diarrhea, febrility, erysipelas, and erythema are of greater importance to it than the diseases for which they are only secondary characteristics. In many respects, an archetypal medicine is forced to be age-old and to continue a tradition from which modern medicine believes it can dissociate itself.

*

He was a graceful young man who often felt cold and therefore most of the time wore a foulard scarf tied artfully around his neck when he came to a psychotherapy session. He sought medical attention for several reasons, not the least of which was that he became ill again and again with colds which were more or less difficult to explain.

The patient's grandfather was an artist who produced predominantly ice-cold paintings, abstract configurations that made it difficult for the viewer to find in them a sympathetic understanding. In his oil paintings, he anticipated a future era of glass and concrete. The patient's father, likewise an artist of glassy coldness, had suffered periodic schizophrenic episodes and finally opened one of his arteries. By contrast, the mother of the patient was afflicted with recurring emotional turmoil; she worried far more than necessary about her son and thereby drove him to desperation.

After his father's death, the patient lived in a small French town with his mother, his grandmother, and an aunt, in a feminine environment that was as frustrating as it was indulgent and overexcited. He suffered vague anxieties about life, often believed himself to be on the verge of a fainting fit, and saw himself as a *quantité négligeable*, a 'negligible quantity,' without any aim or will power. He often thought of opening his carotic artery in order to put an end to his life, but he was much too undecided to carry out his intention. Despite all these inner difficulties, the patient eventually passed his final examinations after attending various middle schools. Thereafter he studied art history, changed his place of residence and his university several times without ever quite knowing what he finally wanted to be. He wandered about in many other ways, too. Because of his attractive appearance, his likable and polite manners, he could easily charm other people; he was a welcome guest on all continents. Everywhere he found opportunities to travel through the world in a parasitical manner and, as a result, a somewhat fraudulent element in his character found sustenance.

Especially at times when he no longer succeeded in getting people interested in him, he was overcome by a particularly chilly emptiness, and he would fall ill with vague fever conditions. Sometimes it was a 'slight cold,' sometimes a regular illness accompanied by fever. Often one did not know what to make of it medically, for the fevers were 'genuine' and held the attention of the worried women. The complicated son always moved at the edge of his physical power of resistance, and a little increase in stress could turn small frustrations into noxious diseases. Physicians who were consulted considered *Roborierung*, a strengthening of the delicate young man, and prescribed medicines to increase his blood pressure, antidepressants to brighten his mood and fortify his ego; they proceeded to purify his blood; they injected multivitamin preparations in order to 'vitalize' his organism; they gave him injections of calcium which, as is well-known, brings about a suggestive warmth during its application.

After ten years of the patient's ailing, the doctors discovered lymph nodes on his neck which became sometimes larger, sometimes smaller. Indeed, after a thorough examination they found a *toxoplasmosis*, a protozoan infection. With great probability the disease had not existed in him before, because previous tests for this condition had proved negative. Rather, it appears as if a more profound chill had searched for a dependable infectious agent that could meet permanently the existential needs of the patient.

Experience has shown that the therapy of toxoplasmosis with sulfonamides is of dubious value. But after about five years, the patient's disease was rendered inactive. During these years psychotherapy was also practiced sporadically, with rather long intervals between sessions. Within this time a great number of questions regarding the temperature of life's climate played an important role, regardless of whether they were expressed or not. Owing to his intelligence, a mercantile cleverness, and an ability to recognize the existential value of warmth and cold more consciously, the patient finally settled down successfully in a border area of the arts, in the fine art trade. Generally he became more resistant and remained largely immune to his fever spells.

*

The coldness in our lives cannot be avoided, and our stress situations are ineluctable. We can no more escape the chills in a gray world than the heat of battle. Goethe's poem is not merely a frightening rural vision, because the white-haired elf-king also travels through the cities with his gray daughters. Emotional cold is an element of life, provided for humankind in the same way as glowing passion, a frozen wintry landscape, or the scorching sun. But it seems as if man must often live at the edge of his thermic frustration tolerance, replacing an insufficient emotional warmth by its somatization—fever. As an individual he falls victim to fever conditions; or in an epidemic he may suffer, along with an immense number of his fellows, an outbreak of influenza in late fall or winter when nature appears mysteriously gloomy, lonely, and empty.

In this context can be placed a pathognomonic dream from which the patient awakened with his characteristic malady of fever:

> I am sitting in the desolate railroad restaurant of a small town. Only a few guests are sitting at the old wooden tables in the half-dark locale. I get up and walk to the counter to get some pastry and liquor. To a colleague, who sees me walking by with my tray, I am saying something like: "I need something to get drunk."[2] Later I find myself atop some modern buildings of the sixties, and as if from an airplane I see to my astonishment a volcano on which snow has fallen and which is standing there all covered with ice. The mountain is illuminated by fabulous moonlight, a cold light in which the bright green of banana bushes stands out in front of the dark, azure-blue sky. I believe that I can hear voices of a party coming from lighted rooms. Suddenly everyone is terrified by a violent detonation, and the volcano ejects gigantic fragments of lava; there is a thundering noise. I see the houses burning, and I want to flee to safety.

A fever attack, as well as those previously mentioned conversions of temperature, appears to be reflected in this icy-fiery scenery. In the first phase the intention—to get drunk in order to get warm—springs from the boredom of a small-town railroad restaurant. It is most admirably understood in the model of a beginning fever represented here that alcohol is everywhere recommended as a preventive and curative remedy against 'colds.' In the second phase, glowing lava breaks out of a silent, ice-covered volcano. The dream points out that a natural occur-

rence such as fever can be understood not only on the personal
level—from the constellation of the family, for example—but
also on the deeper level of an imagination compelled to reach
much further into a place—nature myths, for instance—from
which such a biologicum eventually developed.

*

If in the framework of analysis the susceptibility to fever and
subfebrility stands in the foreground, the conversation will
often turn to themes of heat and cold and their relationship to
each other. These need not actually be sought out, for they appear quite naturally on their own account; the therapy session
is inclined to take this direction as if by itself. It seems as if the
patient's nature wants to avail itself of the analytical conversation to influence that weak resistance, the ever-threatening
Sollverstellung—'adjustment of the normal condition'—by means
of an increasing consciousness. It seems as if the association
with heat and cold needs to be learned by using the detour of
language and the mind in order to break their compelling
powers. The analytical discourse concerning the temperatures
that qualify human existence is thus motivated from rather unconscious regions.

The aim in such cases will be to increase the understanding of
complementary meanings, as in every analytical treatment of a
physical syndrome. Cold is not something that has merely the
connotation of discomfort: to be considered an error of nature,
as it were. And, by the same token, heat does not denote only
good things. On the contrary, these momentary meanings are
highly relative. Just as the stability of nature depends on the
regular interplay of temperatures, 'psychic temperatures' appear
to be determined as well by multifold regulations.

Everything that is generally understood by the concept cold
will scintillate in many ways during therapy. Matters will not
rest merely with complaints about nervousness nor with difficulties in forming relationships and homelessness. Nor will it

be enough to lament the fact that the patient feels himself a stranger everywhere and, misunderstood, placed into an infinite loneliness. There will not only be complaints about lovelessness, about boredom, lack of enthusiasm, and so forth. All this can be interpreted in a different manner; there may be discussion of the ability for a cool fulfillment of one's duty and of the readiness to subject oneself to an abstract task. The conversation may turn to the coldness of pride, to aristocratic distance, to the superior distinction of non-involvement, even to the Far-Eastern philosophic significance of emptiness and nothing. The senselessness or vanity of existence will be a topic of discussion, perhaps also the *Nil Admirari*—'don't admire anything'—of the Stoic doctrine and, above all, the necessity for cold calculation.

While the torment of coldness is thus capable of taking on a particularly intellectual splendor, the value of warmth is also relativized. There will be not only praise for the comforts of home, for the cozy idyll, and a profound mutual understanding; love will not keep its value, and all warming fascination and enthusiasm will lose their sacrosanct importance. Unexpectedly, coziness will become rather dull, and homeyness a life in the dusk of a stable. Love may be related to all manner of blindness. Burning desire may rise like a demon from the abyss, stability may become stagnation, and one will no longer be able to discuss enthusiasm without speaking also of illusion and rapture. Ardent interest will suddenly be nothing but idiotic narrow-mindedness.

*

If we assume that a susceptibility to fever exists wherever psychic warmth is too easily somatized, then in the framework of analytical psychotherapy we will behave as we do when confronted with a 'neurotic symptom.' In such a case, it is a matter of spinning gold from something that apparently has no value, as straw is spun in the tale of Rumpelstiltskin. It is a matter of creating a higher consciousness, of supporting refinements and differentiations, and of recognizing polar values. The analytic treatment of a psychopathological case is not fundamentally different from the treatment of a physical syndrome. An awareness of the reversible significance of everything sick and healthy seems to be an unconditional prerequisite for any guidance and attendance of analytical processes. For how else could their course be protected from all the seductive dangers, possibilities of misrepresentations, and wrong ways, if not by the criterion of paradox, before which all things remain changeable and which, like a magic stone, counteracts torpor and relativizes exaggerations. Knowledge about the ultimately paradoxical meaning of every syndrome is a mental *terra firma*, as it were, the standpoint from which the processes continue—substantial only because it is also chimerical.

Knowledge of the fundamental therapeutic significance of this paradox is by no means new; it was important already in many earlier forms of analytical psychotherapy, not least in alchemical speculation. It is therefore no surprise that alchemy, too, has found symbols for our existence in the contrasts of temperature: Boschius's emblem shows the Mount Etna volcano to be a massive, frozen block ablaze with flames. A meditative contemplation of such a paradoxical *philosophem* best illustrates our analytical concern with a syndrome like fever.

1. Even in the history of language the concept "fever" scintillates between cold and warm. On the one hand, the Indo-Germanic root *preus* becomes the Latin *pruino* 'hoar-frost,' as an ice-coating over objects; and in several other languages, it develops into words meaning things similar to "frost." On the other, the Latin *prurire* 'burning,' 'itching' or *pruna* 'the glowing coal' can be traced back to the same root, as can also the Old Indian *prusto* 'scorched'; and the Latin words *febris* 'the fever,' *fovere* 'to warm,' and *favilla* 'glowing ashes' are linguistically related to the Middle High German *friezen* 'the fever,' *frörer* 'to freeze,' and to today's *Fraisen*, 'the feverish convulsions of children.'
2. [Translator's note: these words are English in the original.]

The Hydrolith
On Drinking and Dryness

I

AN archetypal understanding of man and his diseases lies beyond the realm of logic. Although in the course of the history of the humanities many attempts have been made, none has really dealt in earnest with the archetypal standpoint. Traditional or, as Kant termed it, classical logic which unites the natural sciences is not at all suited for this task, for the 'archetypal' cannot be dealt with according to the principles of identity or contradiction, nor does it maintain a legitimate relationship to the principle of cause and effect, i.e., to causality.

Despite all attempts to at least hybridize archetypal reflection and logic, the former eludes our grasp again and again. It seems from the very beginning to be of a basically different nature and in many respects to complement logic. Communion with the archetypal is unique and wakens in us sensations which are much more 'sophical' than 'logical.' Archetypal understanding is, in fact, a communion with *sophia* 'wisdom,' rather than with *logos*, 'intelligence' in the narrower sense of the word. It seems as if we were dealing with two different forms of intellectual eros, and we may wonder, on first hearing the word "sophical" and on fathoming its true significance, that it has heretofore been missing from our vocabulary.

This must be due to the one-sided presuppositions of our culture. Actually, the pre-Socratics had already diagnosed our intellectual dichotomy. It seems to have been Heraclitus who first introduced the word *philosophos*, which he used to differentiate those who loved wisdom from those who were 'only' intellectuals. In the later works of Plato, the philosopher becomes characterized by his modesty, knowing that he knows nothing while remaining enthralled by his love of wisdom. In the works of Aristotle, communion with sophia becomes the *prima philosophia* or metaphysics in the proper sense. The Romans also made the existential distinction between *sapientia* 'wisdom' and *scientia* 'science.' This is not the place to further explore this differentiation. Nonetheless, we may ascertain with astonishment that the majority of the philosophers were not philosophers at all but rather philologists, for they were concerned almost exclusively with logos; hence their spirits loved a different sphere.

Even on the bare experimental level, communion with the archetypal appears to be something special, and this continues to hold true on other levels. Thinking becomes more contemplative; in the place of clearly defined concepts, we encounter iridescence or even twilight. What is lost in clarity and precision is exchanged for an increase in depth. When the 'superficial' bond to time and space becomes of secondary importance, then eternity steps into the foreground, and development is superseded by the eternal present. What is lost in the earthshaking practicability of logical concepts is retrieved in 'magic.' What is missing in cerebral insights is replaced by empathy. Such contemplation is a function of the entire body. Whatever had been logically perspicuous now becomes urgent and passionate. And whenever serious distress would otherwise prevail, in matters of life and death, we encounter drama, whereby our existence takes on a quasi-illusory quality introducing irony. Archetypal understanding ranges in the realm of the possible, it is 'possibilistic,' and its language is not that of the scientist but that of the poet who muses.

*

Hence, if analytical psychology strives for an archetypal understanding of man and his suffering, we discover two obscurities and an unjustified modesty in the nomenclature. First, as we have demonstrated above, it has very little to do with '-logy' and is, properly speaking, in no way comparable to that which other sciences utilizing this suffix pursue. The association studies marked the historical conclusion of that part of Jung's work which can be considered to belong to the realm of conventional science. Everything that came later was born of a different spirit and was much more a courting of wisdom. This new position, however, seems to have been so misleadingly formulated that to the present day attempts at a retroactive corruption are made again and again. It seems to me that new attempts are constantly being made to integrate analytical psychology —tying it down by force—into the currently official scientific framework.

Second, after my introductory remarks concerning logos and sophia, one can hardly speak of analytical psychology as being analytic, because analysis means 'the resolution or dissection of one into many.' One might sooner refer to it as being synthetic, but even then one would imply a construction and unification that was not intended. It might be more accurately termed the art of interpreting primal images, because it proceeds from specific phenomena via a primarily analogical path to the archetypal, thereby revealing meaning. It is an art, not a technique.

Third and finally, analytical psychology imposes upon itself a limitation which I have to this day never been able to understand: although it is characterized by its communion with the archetypal, it purports, at least nominally, not to deal with the entire person, the *anthropos*, but rather to limit itself to his 'psyche.' Although it would be natural for analytical psychology to be a general pathosophy, whereby every analytical psychologist would as a matter of course be considered a physician, it restricts itself instead to psychiatry. Hence it isolates the soul as a 'relatively closed system,' separating it from the entirety of the person and bringing archetypal reflection to bear on it. Then it becomes necessary to reconnect the body and the soul via more or less plausible mental gymnastics. One speaks, for example, of the 'irradiation' of the psychic into the somatic, etc. However benevolent and willing we may be, we are stuck with a theoretical scandal.

Aside from the element of illogic, it is probably this curious self-restriction to dealing with the psyche which has led analytical psychology to have so little intercourse with medicine. If ever someone should fall prey to the desire to bring order into the diversity of physical illness using analytical psychology, he would soon give up in despair. Medical experience cannot be integrated into analytical psychology, not only because the latter is illogical but also because it has not applied archetypal reflection to the whole person.

And so it is that we succumb to fictions. It is as if in therapy we could conduct a pseudo-business without consulting one of the partners. By concerning ourselves with psychic behavior and leaving the body to the technicians, because it does not belong to the relatively closed system of the psyche, we move in a dimension that is variously sustained by another one without this being adequately realized. Or do we really take adequately into account how closely the disappearance of psychic syndromes may correspond to the development of more or less evident physical illness? The question is not meant moralistically but rather from the standpoint of the theory of cognition. It is apparently not possible to do justice to all sides simultaneously. But it does seem that the exclusion of bodily pathology would encourage us to move in an unreal world of the so-called psychic.

*

Archetypal understanding of man and his suffering did not originate in the twentieth century. On the contrary, we can trace it throughout the whole of occidental intellectual history.

But it is as if this were only a sort of *via occulta*, a dark path which runs in the shadow of the official sciences. It is as if everyone who tread this path were something of an outsider. They were termed either heathens or heretics and were excommunicated or burned at the stake by the Church. An archetypal understanding was not easily integrated with the spirit which, among other things, produced our concept of the highest sacred value, the Christian God. It can be appended neither to a unipolar, unchangeable Creator nor to His image and likeness, *homo faber*, who always remains identical with himself while creating the 'best of all possible worlds.' Compared to this, the primary characteristics of archetypal understanding seem to me to be of a dramatically different nature.

Historically, this becomes most apparent in reference to completely different concepts of God and man, namely, when the highest being is an eternally changing figure, pantheistic, and simultaneously the world and, as such, subject to suffering due to inner conflicts. Naturally this is correlated to a similar image of man as monadic, changeable, and subject to suffering. And just as the Creator is linked to *homo faber* by their similarity and communion, there is also a correspondence between macrocosmos and microcosmos and a participation of the one in the other. In the case of the changeable deity, one is tempted to see not a male but a female godhead and image of man. This conjures up not only visions of the gods of India and the Far East but even more importantly the experience of a realliance with sophia as wisdom.

To arbitrarily commence an arbitrary historical enumeration, such an understanding of god and man is already discernible among the pre-Socratics. For example, the enigmatic Heraclitus held the world to be a god struggling with eruptions of elemental passions or actually of a world-fire in which manifestations arise and disappear again. The sequel to this image may be found in Plato, where the eternal fire becomes an intelligent unchanging deity who manifests himself in the diversity of the

world and who has a central heart similar to that postulated by
Pythagoras. The suffering but also spectral world then becomes
his theater. This primary Platonic insight takes on another form
in late Neoplatonism and in the Platonism of the Florentine
renaissance. The latter may have inspired Shakespeare to hang
the motto "totus mundus agit histrionem" ('all the world's a
stage') over the entrance to the Globe Theater. If we exclude the
baroque period, which tends anyway to be world-theater, we
find that archetypal understanding takes on new forms during
the romantic period. 'Primordial phenomena' take on a thousand changing forms, and the god whom they constitute
becomes a monstrous organism which is kept in motion by the
struggle of its inner contradictions. This image corresponds to
the unstable and passionate romantic personality who anticipated an increase in the intensity of his existential experience to accrue particularly from the asthenic, from multiple
illness. Such a figure never seems to be completely in earnest
and always has a touch of irony about him, going through life
"trembling and tottering" as Novalis put it.

Thus, wherever in the history of the humanities we meet with
an understanding that gives preference to the archetypal, we
will encounter notions and a language which are, so to speak,
those of Nature herself. They are not cerebral but rather bodily
and emotionally moving.

*

After this digression into the history of religion I would like to
develop a more detailed discussion of the three characteristics,
mentioned above, which especially characterize the archetypal.
Though there are certainly more such characteristics, these will
suffice to clarify what is meant by the term "archetypal
medicine," which will be examined more closely in the second
part of my paper. Although these characteristics seem to be
independent of one another, they almost always appear in conjunction with one another, as we have just seen in our digres-

sion on the history of religion. Nonetheless, in cognitive theory they constitute separate units. We will be considering: the mutability of the archetypal, the fact that it most often reveals itself as pairs of opposites, and its relatedness to a central focus.

First, the *mutability*, or *changeableness*, of the archetypal manifests itself in archetypal medicine most strikingly when behavior is transformed into a physical gestalt and vice versa. What was recently an aspect of demeanor can be transformed and appear as a physical symptom. Hence our readiness to be shaken or moved can be transformed into a physical trembling disease, our reluctance can appear more or less abruptly in different forms of rheumatic stiffness, or our ability to keep life moist may reappear in addiction to water and edema. Such embodiments operate like the inferior function of analytical psychology: they too lead to some of the most difficult complications in life, especially when they sink below a level that would previously have just been tolerable.

Hence, the archetypal alters only its appearance. It searches, so to speak, for another aggregate condition, condenses, immobilizes, or even makes one bedridden. The basic psychosomatic question, namely, how psychic phenomena influence the body, hardly even arises. The archetypal already belongs to a dimension that is sufficiently broad to allow such metamorphoses to take place. In addition, the boundaries that separate the so-called functional from truly organic disturbances are clouded. What would otherwise enmesh the diagnostician in punctilious argumentation becomes a question of the depth of somatization from the archetypal point of view. What arise are more or less reversible, mutable syndromes (images of illness) which ought not to be confused with units of disease. The latter derive from another form of medicine, that of the natural sciences. It has been my experience that mixing the two uncritically leads to annoying difficulties in communication. One must stick to the 'images' and wonder at the sometimes so astonishing dramatics of which Nature is capable.

Second, the archetypal tends to *appear as opposites*. It is as if a need for a more rigidly structured understanding were being thereby satisfied, for with all its changeability the world tends to get out of bounds. Hence, one finds awe more or less openly affiliated with arrogance, inflexibility with compliance, and preference for the wet with a longing for the dry. There is nothing final or stable in the relationship between the opposites, but rather it is a diverse dialectic which proves to be the rule. Sometimes a complementarity of the opposites may awaken the impression of a special harmony; at other times, one is faced with almost indistinguishable contortions, or with a blur or, finally, a mutual avoidance, equivalent to an inner rift, may be the case, inducing on the one hand inflation and on the other somatization. Thus, the archetypal tends not only to pull us completely into its sphere and to impose an absolute and exclusive style upon us but also to condemn its complement to bodily exile, where it is then compelled to lead a demoralized, often surreal existence. The occasion of such a metamorphosis is most often an aporetic moment of being trapped without an alternative. This occurs when life has taken on bizarre proportions.

Finally, the archetypal strives for structure not only in the polarization mentioned above, but even more it tends to be related to *a virtual center*. It is as if it were constantly oriented around this center, like the pantheistic deities around a world-navel. Hence, all of the dialectic variations of the relationships of the archetypal, as well as their above-mentioned potential for metamorphosis, maintain at all times a point of reference. It is as if our life followed a golden thread of meaning, despite the fact that we may have to confront extremes of repulsion, nothingness, and absurdity. Whether we like it or not, Nature compels us to a 'philosophical life' in the sense defined above: we cannot avoid a lifelong desire for sophia, the wisdom that lets all the horrible variations of Being be encountered as something numinous and amazing.

II

In this section, I would like to try to interpolate the topics of thirst and drinking and their morbid alterations into the general theory of archetypal medicine which I have briefly sketched. We are going to have to pose the same fundamental question which was originally raised by Heraclitus, i.e., how does that which is liquid, wet, or moist relate to that which is dry or, in the language of the pre-Socratics, what does Dionysos have to do with Hades?

It may be said that wetness and moisture introduce chaos, are inclined to intoxication and delirium. Hence, according to the Taoists, water can have no boundaries, because wetness harbors chasms and infinity. Considering water's dangerousness, Isaiah besought the Lord to rescue him, because the waters of death had penetrated his soul, and he was drowning in filth. On the other hand, wetness also harbors genius, originality, and humor. (In German the word for salvation is even etymologically related to hydrophysics—*Erlösung: Lösung* means 'solution.') The positive aspect of water is why Christ could say that he would give drink to the thirsty, that water would fall in the desert and springs would open up in the land of thirst and make it fertile. That is also why the Holy Spirit completes Christ's redemptive work as the *fons vivus*, pouring down on mankind as a living spring.

Indeed, Dionysos and Bacchus are closely related to wetness and fluids. They are the gods of the instinctive and the driven. It is they who tend toward motility, delirium, swelling, and decomposition. But it is also their spirit which inspires the arts, which brings the world comedies and tragedies and laughter, and which in the orphic-bacchic mysteries promises redemption from life through life itself.

Dryness, on the other hand, tends toward infertility, sterility, endless frustration, renunciation, and privation. According to the history of symbols, it is not only salty but also bitter; as dust it has the meaning of nothingness. On the other hand, dryness enjoys the highest respect as that through which everything arises out of the flood of the indistinguishable. So it was that in the story of the creation the first "Let there be . . ." called forth dryness, the first firmament. In Tantrism the ego is composed of dryness and thereby differentiates itself from a universal Being, and in the Bible the drunkard Noah sees it as the land of the future. In alchemical speculation, many islands combine to compose a standpoint much as sparks combine to form the light of consciousness. Dryness reminds one of the asceticism of the inner world, of puritanism, of an urbanity which we try to preserve with a plethora of fire, i.e., of energy.

Indeed, it resembles Hades who takes after his father Cronus, who ate his children, inasmuch as Hades tends to destroy life. Not only does he not even look at or listen to life, his head being on backwards, but he also causes it to decompose and disappear and makes himself and others invisible, thereby taking away their vital energy. In this respect, he is similar to the Christian 'death' who, in the form of a rattling, bone-dry skeleton, reaps the living with his scythe. In contrast to Dionysos, Hades turns an ominous visage to the world; he is a stern deity. Accordingly, he inhabits a desolate, rocky, dusty Tartarus where dusk never really gives way to light. Although several rivers run through Tartarus, an endless desert of sand and stone seems to stretch out there, and one encounters everywhere frustrated souls tortured by thirst. One encounters, of course, also the dastardly Danaides, who hopelessly try to fill a barrel which is full of holes, and the degenerate Tantalus, who fruitlessly tries to quench his thirst with the water in which he is standing.

Still this unhappy picture does have a lighter side—when Hades becomes Pluto and as such possessor of chthonic wealth in the form of all sorts of jewels and metals. He is closely related to scientific artfulness and technical processing and was hence in Rome termed simply 'Dis,' the rich man. Hades must be somehow related to our urban civilization and to the modern, rational coming of age. The more we exclude death from our lives, the more it spreads ubiquitously in the form of a general, gray, stony urbanity.

*

It is certain that all of us are in one way or another and to one degree or another determined by dionysian tendencies and by the dryness of Hades. But it is often not so easy to distinguish the two and to separate their spheres of influence. We are then subject to a well-known predicament, just as we are liable to become bewildered by the polarized iridescence of the psychic attitudes and functions. There we get into the same difficulty of not being able to state with certainty which is really the dominant and which the inferior function. Often we can only establish that this life is marked by this or that conflict.

When the functions can be determined, experience has proved that it is the darker of the two, the so-called inferior function, which not only provokes psychic trouble but also tends to be *embodied* (transformed into a physical illness). The latter happens, as we have already mentioned, when the dominant function takes too unquestioned possession of us. Hence, when dryness in one form or another sets the keynote to our life, we can expect that a neglected 'drunkenness on life' will show itself as an illness in which exceptional thirst and compulsive drinking play a role. What was previously visible only as a psychic disequilibrium becomes more and more distorted and begins to extend into the realm of physical medicine.

*

A whole range of more or less serious illnesses through which Dionysos can overtake us originates in this manner. We may well all understand that we reach for a glass when we have run dry. This otherwise unremarkable act can reach the intensity of an awful need for certain persons who—as it is phrased in psychosomatic literature—are of dry, nervous susceptibility. They may be compelled to drink up to twenty liters of fluids daily. Then it is very difficult to determine to what degree physical alterations are a contributing factor, e.g., whether the production of the hormones which regulate the metabolism of fluids is disturbed perhaps by brain damage due to an encephalitis or to a tumor which affects areas of the brain stem. We will be speaking presently of diabetes insipidus, though it is uncertain whether Nature goes so far as to somatize to that extent.

There are also forms of alcoholism, especially beer drinking, which are linked to a disturbance in the regulation of fluids. It is then often easy to establish that the patients are driven to drink and to become bloated by their exceptional sobriety and boredom, i.e., by their 'thirsty souls.'

Thirst and the compulsion to drink can become especially torturing for diabetics who are also said to be prone to a dry performance of their duties and to choleric self-frustration. When untreated, diabetes insipidus can also lead to bloating.

*

In related syndromes, 'drunkenness on life' is somatized and develops into a monstrous drinking bout. We shrink, so to speak, to something inorganic, but in doing so we succumb to a process that is not other than that which takes place in most illnesses. The environment of the rheumatic patient becomes less 'lively' when his resistance embodies itself in his joints, as does the environment of the skin patient when his need for isolation takes on the form of reptilian scales, or of the trembler who must experience being deeply moved as a tremor. Last but not least, the lonely psychotic becomes a 'case' when the enzyme secretion of his brain goes its own way and he hallucinates his relationship to the world.

Our environment not only becomes inorganic as we do but also bizarre. Normally the organism maintains certain concentrations and dilutions throughout the body. In and between the cells, there is an optimal saturation, i.e., a balanced relationship among all sorts of salts—especially chloric and sugar salts—and their solvent, water. This balance belongs, so to speak, to our genetic inheritance from the time of our prehistoric, oceanic origins. We live best at a certain level of aqueousness, with an optimal tumescence. It is as if Nature were in this respect subject to a *horror torri* 'a fear of drying up.' In diseases of thirst, however, the dry salts, following the laws of osmotic wedlock, carry the water off in enormous quantities of urine or draw it into the body tissue, so that a compulsive but futile drinking is the result. Thirst is then located not only in a burning, fevery throat. The osmotic catastrophe is rather a torture of general insatiability.

*

This change is terrible and purports a mythic destiny. It reminds one in many ways of bacchic dipsomania and of some traditions concerning the diseases of Dionysos. Without forcing the issue, one may include here the fate of Tantalus, king of the Phrygians. As is well-known, he suffers eternal thirst in the Hades of the Greeks for having stolen sweet nectar from the table of the gods. It is as if archaic fantasy had tried to explain diabetes in this fashion, just as the collective imagination in general, of course, attempts to enmesh the sick person in the web of serious tales. There are similar legends in the Germanic culture.

There, however, Tantalus becomes a devilish figure called the 'eternal thirst.' He in turn is related to Wodan who was truly the god of drunkenness. Not only mead but also the arts of poetry and music belong to his domain. He is a figure similar to the Mediterranean Dionysos. But he was also a god of warmaking that had little to do with technique and much to do with the love of fighting, killing, and the blood-curdling. It was not so long ago that he raced on stormy nights with his dead warriors through remote valleys in the highlands of Switzerland. But it is as if *he* too were not only banned from the new religions but had also, as was the case with Bacchus and Tantalus, retreated to the world of pathology. It is as if he not only haunted our rational era like a shadow but had also incarnated himself in various illnesses where hardly anyone recognizes him.

Wodan is also called *Türst* in Switzerland, and *Türse* is an archaic term for giants. It is a manifold relationship. They too are characterized as humid and ecstatic. According to the legends, they not only brewed thunderstorms in huge kettles, but they were also nursed for seven years. Their drunkenness was well-known, and they were seen toasting to one another across the mountains. They were never very clever and—like Wodan who, as reason and enlightenment took over the land, had to retreat to the remoter regions and to withdraw into the realm of illness—they too had to embody themselves, though it is said that they all were conquered 'full of wine' in a war against the cunning Austrians.

It is notable, of course, that everywhere reference could be made to the disturbance of the hormonal secretions that regulate the balance of fluids and salts we mentioned above. There is in fact an endocrine psycho-syndrome, a more or less characteristic personality change accompanying hormonal diseases. It is characterized particularly by drive and need disturbances, by mood swings, etc. It occurs in acromegaly and in acromegalic growth disturbances where one can see a tendency to giantism in the extremities—the hands, feet, chin, and nose. This is often accompanied by excesses of all sorts, including in drinking.

*

For centuries, whenever drinking has become a compulsion and the disease of thirst has taken on a medical dimension because the individual has gotten too dried up, treatment has centered around the question of how much wetness and dryness were beneficial for the patient. It becomes an attempt to influence the osmotic relationship, and the ambivalent affair has provided the opportunity for the most diverse and contradictory prescriptions. There is a long history of dispute over the therapy of osmotic conditions: over, on the one hand, what quantities of salts, of carbohydrates which are turned into salts, and of proteins which retain water, etc. and, on the other hand, what quantities of daily fluids can be prescribed for the patient.

The treatment always follows one of two ancient therapeutic principles: on the one hand, a drying out according to the principle of *contrarium contrario* was felt to be necessary. One *countered* it, because everything monstrous calls opposing forces into play. Deprivation of fluids and dry food were prescribed, although this led in some cases to death accompanied by tortures of thirst. Sweating was prescribed, or the patients were sent to the desert. On the other hand, it was held that *similis simile curatur*, and the opposite was done. One acquiesced to the desire, prescribed drinking and bathing, and the thirsty diabetics traveled to the famous baths at Karlsbad and Vichy.

Today the treatment of compulsive drinking is certainly more effective. In addition to the appropriate diet, there are diuretics, substances which remove the salts and hence the concomitant water from the body. Or hormones, like insulin, are prescribed, which play a role in the regulation of the osmotic balance.

Despite all pragmatic doctoring, one feels nonetheless the necessity of *orienting our actions toward the archetypal*. The treatment remains insufficient if it is performed only with the ingenuity of the natural sciences and remains puerile despite all its diversity and effectiveness. From the beginning, a philosophical standpoint obtrudes upon us and requires of both physician and patient a contemplation of the archetypal in fluids and in dry things, because their conflict is so fateful. It is as if we, despite all the therapy, would not otherwise know where we stand. Nature does not take well to being understood and treated solely on the basis of rational knowledge or from a social particular disposition, it also awakens a *particular* numinous sensation. Contemplating it lets us begin to sense that frustration, self-discipline, and rationality, on the one hand, and satisfaction and art, on the other, are related in a manner that is at once mysterious and sober. Reflecting on the Hydrolith may clarify for us how to approach Dionysos and Hades. It contains a philo-sophical knowledge of how much privation and redemption may await us in this life. This may not only help preventive medicine to prevent the outbreak of the maladies we have been considering but also to bring about an inner stability when they have already reached the point where they are irreversible and lead to death.

Also from Spring Publications on Illness and Therapy

Masochism
Lyn Cowan

Lyn Cowan, a practicing Jungian analyst, stresses the symptoms of masochism, which range from the kinkiest of sexual aberrations to the covert pleasure felt in the minor hurts and humiliations of ordinary life, and reads them both as signs of an actual sickness and as stirrings of the collective psyche. Included is a thorough discussion of the clinical literature—Krafft-Ebing, Freud, etc.—as well as cultural case studies, the Flagellants of medieval times. Regarded here as a manifestation of the religious instinct, masochism emerges as a strange necessity of the psyche that can lead the reader deeper into the pleasure and pain of his or her own vulnerabilities, there to discover the germ of genuine individuality. (137 pgs.)

Eros on Crutches
Adolf Guggenbühl-Craig

The author takes up the most frightening shadow of our times: not the violent street criminal but the decay in morality that allows psychopathy to live close by without recognition. Today we can hardly see the psychopath or our own psychopathic traits. Guggenbühl evokes sympathy for this figure even as he explores his radical defects of character summed up in his inability to experience Eros. In the psychopath's soul Eros is on crutches. (126 pgs.)

Echo's Subtle Body
Patricia Berry

Collected here, all of Patricia Berry's writings between 1972 and 1982 together develop a style of psychotherapy based on the primacy of the image in psychical life. The book contains the often mentioned but long out-of-print "An Approach to the Dream" and "What's the Matter with Mother," as well as the new papers, "The Dogma of Gender" and "The Shadow of Training/The Training of Shadow." The insights bolstered by clinical example, dream interpretation, and mythical references, each paper revisions an important analytic construct—reduction, dream, defense, *telos* or goal, reflection, shadow—so that it more adequately echoes the poetic basis of mind. (198 pgs.)

Psyche and Death
Edgar Herzog

In this two-part study—first presented as lectures at the C. G. Jung Institute in Zürich—the author attends the Death Image; with skill and care he exhumes from fairytale and folklore the macabre variations of this most ancient symbol. In such chapters as "Killing" and "The Death-Demon as Fate," Herzog examines the Death Images of archaic humanity, showing that Death originally revealed itself in the guise of an animal: as a Wolf, Horse, Dog, Snake, and Bird. Today Death takes similar forms but appears to human consciousness mainly through dreams instead of via myth and ritual. In Part Two, Herzog focuses on the dreams of patients in psychotherapy and glosses those dreams with remarkable interpretations that link their persons, scenes, and drama to the symbolic images and rites of the ancient past. (224 pgs.)

The Book of Life
Marsilio Ficino

The first translation ever in English of this underground classic of the Italian Renaissance, a book once suppressed for Ficino's approach to images, daemons, and planets in relation to health. In a fluent, amusing, and exact translation by Charles Boer, this founding text of archetypal psychology is a guide to food, drink, sleep, mood, sexuality, song, and countless herbal and vegetable concoctions for maintaining the right balance of soul, body, and spirit. (217 pgs.)

Spring Publications, Inc. • P.O. Box 222069 • Dallas, Texas 75222